# Epidemics and Pandemics

## *Your Questions Answered*

Charles Vidich

BLOOMSBURY ACADEMIC
NEW YORK • LONDON • OXFORD • NEW DELHI • SYDNEY

BLOOMSBURY ACADEMIC
Bloomsbury Publishing Inc
1385 Broadway, New York, NY 10018, USA
50 Bedford Square, London, WC1B 3DP, UK
29 Earlsfort Terrace, Dublin 2, Ireland

BLOOMSBURY, BLOOMSBURY ACADEMIC and the Diana logo are
trademarks of Bloomsbury Publishing Plc

First published in the United States of America 2024

A catalog record for this book is available from the Library of Congress.

ISBN:   HB:   978-1-4408-8138-1
       ePDF:  978-1-4408-8139-8
       eBook:  979-8-7651-1048-5

Series: Q&A Health Guides

Typeset by Integra Software Services Pvt. Ltd.
Printed and bound in Great Britain

To find out more about our authors and books visit www.bloomsbury.com
and sign up for our newsletters.

# Epidemics and Pandemics

# Contents

# Series Foreword

All of us have questions about our health. Is this normal? Should I be doing something differently? Whom should I talk to about my concerns? And our modern world is full of answers. Thanks to the Internet, there's a wealth of information at our fingertips, from forums where people can share their personal experiences to Wikipedia articles to the full text of medical studies. But finding the right information can be an intimidating and difficult task—some sources are written at too high a level, others have been oversimplified, while still others are heavily biased or simply inaccurate.

*Q&A Health Guides* address the needs of readers who want accurate, concise answers to their health questions, authored by reputable and objective experts, and written in clear and easy-to-understand language. This series focuses on the topics that matter most to young adult readers, including various aspects of physical and emotional well-being as well as other components of a healthy lifestyle. These guides will also serve as a valuable tool for parents, school counselors, and others who may need to answer teens' health questions.

All books in the series follow the same format to make finding information quick and easy. Each volume begins with an essay on health literacy and why it is so important when it comes to gathering and evaluating health information. Next, the top five myths and misconceptions that surround the topic are dispelled. The heart of each guide is a collection of questions and answers, organized thematically. A selection of five case studies provides real-world examples to illuminate key concepts. Rounding out each volume are a directory of resources, glossary, and index.

It is our hope that the books in this series will not only provide valuable information but will also help guide readers toward a lifetime of healthy decision making.

# Acknowledgments

Authoring this book required the emotional and intellectual support of a team of friends and family who encouraged me with their comments and critiques with earlier drafts of this book. I am indebted to my wife Clare for reading and, in many cases, listening to me read the case studies and question and answer sections of this book. When stories are told aloud, they convey more than mere words—feelings and pauses add to the experience. The feedback I received from editor Maxine Taylor was invaluable to the creation of this book. Her suggestions were spot on, and her encouragement was invaluable as I worked on a tight timetable. This book was a labor of love that builds on over twenty years of research I conducted on the causes of epidemics and the role of quarantine in controlling communicable disease. I am indebted to my nephew Josh Vidich and my sons Jamie and Paul Vidich for taking the time to review earlier versions of the five case studies. Their editorial skills honed through their careers in the publishing world helped immeasurably.

# Introduction

Imagine a wildfire starting where drought conditions have existed for years. The kindling needs less than a match to burst into flames. Within minutes flames can spread hundreds of feet and within days consume thousands of square miles of forest, human settlements, and even subterranean root systems. The flames and heat give immediate warning to all those in the path of the raging inferno. Flee as they may try, many people die, even though no such options exist for the earthbound trees that hold this earth in place. Epidemics are like wildfires except they are far more deadly because their causative factors—bacteria, viruses, and other microbial pathogens—are invisible to the eye and infect humans even without their knowledge. Pandemics are wildfires on steroids and are made worse when the carriers of pandemic disease reveal no outward signs of sickness. Asymptomatic carriers of Covid-19 spread this viral disease even before the heat and flames of the disease (i.e., the Covid-19 symptoms) burst into public view. Our fight or flight instincts are not activated when there is no wildfire to be seen by the naked eye. Yet this is what makes epidemics and pandemics so dangerous.

Covid-19 was a wakeup call for the planet. Americans had not seen a pandemic in the previous 100 years and grew content that medical science had conquered communicable disease. Unbeknownst to many people, highly communicable diseases have quickly adapted to modern antibiotics and antiviral medicines and have become resistant. These superbugs are not the only issue. In a world where every part of the planet can be reached in a matter of hours by plane, the reservoirs of disease in remote regions of the world are now as great a concern for public health as the sickness of our next-door neighbor. Pathogens are getting more resistant to medicine, travel times are shorter, and people are living in much more crowded conditions than fifty years ago. Epidemics are fueled by these enabling factors. However, this book explores far more than the mere enabling conditions that make epidemics and pandemics possible.

The stress and depression that afflicts millions of Americans is made worse during epidemics. This is not a new phenomenon. Epidemics have not only decimated lives they have altered the trajectory of civilizations and the values of cultures. This book reviews the consequences of past and current epidemics and their impacts on public health using an easy-to-read question and answer format so the reader can jump to the specific issues of greatest interest. The questions and answers are interrelated so you can follow ideas from one question to another based on your specific concerns.

The study of epidemics and pandemics has been a concern for every generation for time out of mind. However, unlike previous investigations and research by scientists and public health professionals in the era before the internet and before DNA and RNA genotyping capabilities existed, we are now approaching an era where our scientific and technical skills have accomplished miracles in the fields of laboratory testing and virtual real-time vaccine development. Yet this book explains that our pride is these innovative developments masks a wide range of organizational and behavioral psychology challenges that fail to keep pace with scientific developments.

This book does not sugar coat the challenges of stopping future pandemics. It also does not suggest it will be easy to develop coordinated and consistent approaches to epidemic and pandemic response measures in a multi-cultural democratic society with strong fault lines created by political divides and massive disinformation campaigns.

This book explores the history of epidemics, their causes and countermeasures, and the impacts they have on human behavior. It also addresses the weaknesses of the current regulatory and organizational structures that exist to stop future epidemics and how they work and where they don't. Our ability to beat back the raging inferno of pandemic disease requires a revamped public health system that tempers the command-and-control paradigm. In its place we need to develop a unified incident command system analogous to that used by the US Forest Service to effectively fight wildfires across a wide range of governmental jurisdictions. This is a tall order for a democracy where public health decision-making is primarily the domain of state governments. Yet no one has bothered to inform our ever-present microbial pathogens to stay within the boundaries of state or federal authorities that exist in America. The choice is ours to make; we can fight epidemics single-handedly or we can work across state and international lines in a collaborative multi-jurisdictional approach. This book explores best practices critical to pandemic prevention and response as well as the misconceptions and myths that stand in the way.

# Guide to Health Literacy

On her thirteenth birthday, Samantha was diagnosed with type 2 diabetes. She consulted her mom and her aunt, both of whom also have type 2 diabetes, and decided to go with their strategy of managing diabetes by taking insulin. As a result of participating in an after-school program at her middle school that focused on health literacy, she learned that she can help manage the level of glucose in her bloodstream by counting her carbohydrate intake, following a diabetic diet, and exercising regularly. But, what exactly should she do? How does she keep track of her carbohydrate intake? What is a diabetic diet? How long should she exercise and what type of exercise should she do? Samantha is a visual learner, so she turned to her favorite source of media, YouTube, to answer these questions. She found videos from individuals around the world sharing their experiences and tips, doctors (or at least people who have "Dr." in their YouTube channel names), government agencies such as the National Institutes of Health, and even video clips from cat lovers who have cats with diabetes. With guidance from the librarian and the health and science teachers at her school, she assessed the credibility of the information in these videos and even compared their suggestions to some of the print resources that she was able to find at her school library. Now, she knows exactly how to count her carbohydrate level, how to prepare and follow a diabetic diet, and how much (and what) exercise is needed daily. She intends to share her findings with her mom and her aunt, and now she wants to create a chart that summarizes what she has learned that she can share with her doctor.

Samantha's experience is not unique. She represents a shift in our society; an individual no longer views himself or herself as a passive recipient of medical care but as an active mediator of his or her own health. However, in this era when any individual can post his or her opinions and experiences with a particular health condition online with just a few clicks or publish a memoir, it is vital that people know how to assess the credibility of health information. Gone are the days when "publishing" health information required intense vetting. The health information landscape is highly saturated, and people have innumerable sources where they can find information about practically any health topic. The sources (whether print, online, or a person) that an individual consults for health information are crucial because the accuracy and trustworthiness of the information can potentially affect his or her overall health. The ability to find, select, assess, and use health information constitutes a type of literacy—health literacy—that everyone must possess.

## The Definition and Phases of Health Literacy

One of the most popular definitions for health literacy comes from Ratzan and Parker (2000), who describe health literacy as "the degree to which individuals have the capacity to obtain, process, and understand basic health information and services needed to make appropriate health decisions." Recent research has extrapolated health literacy into health literacy bits, further shedding light on the multiple phases and literacy practices that are embedded within the multifaceted concept of health literacy. Although this research has focused primarily on online health information seeking, these health literacy bits are needed to successfully navigate both print and online sources. There are six phases of health information seeking: (1) Information Need Identification and Question Formulation, (2) Information Search, (3) Information Comprehension, (4) Information Assessment, (5) Information Management, and (6) Information Use.

The first phase is the *information need identification and question formulation phase*. In this phase, one needs to be able to develop and refine a range of questions to frame one's search and understand relevant health terms. In the second phase, *information search*, one has to possess appropriate searching skills, such as using proper keywords and correct spelling in search terms, especially when using search engines and databases. It is also crucial to understand how search engines work (i.e., how search results are derived, what the order of the search results means, how to use the snippets that are provided in the search results list to select websites, and how to determine which listings are ads on a search engine results page). One also has to limit reliance on surface characteristics, such as the design of a website or a book (a website or book that appears to have a lot of information or looks aesthetically pleasant does not necessarily mean it has good information) and language used (a website or book that utilizes jargon, the keywords that one used to conduct the search, or the word "information" does not necessarily indicate it will have good information). The next phase is *information comprehension*, whereby one needs to have the ability to read, comprehend, and recall the information (including textual, numerical, and visual content) one has located from the books and/or online resources.

To assess the credibility of health information (*information assessment phase*), one needs to be able to evaluate information for accuracy, evaluate how current the information is (e.g., when a website was last updated or when a book was published), and evaluate the creators of the source—for example, examine site sponsors or type of sites (.com, .gov, .edu, or .org) or the author of a book (practicing doctor, a celebrity doctor, a patient of a specific disease, etc.) to determine the believability of the person/organization providing the information. Such credibility perceptions tend to become generalized, so they must be frequently reexamined (e.g., the belief that a specific news agency always has credible health information needs continuous vetting). One also needs to evaluate the credibility of the medium (e.g., television, Internet, radio, social media, and book) and evaluate—not just accept without questioning—others' claims regarding the validity of a site, book, or other specific source of information. At this stage, one has to "make sense of information gathered from diverse sources by identifying misconceptions, main and supporting ideas, conflicting information, point of view, and biases" (American Association of School Librarians [AASL], 2009, p. 13) and conclude which sources/information are valid and accurate by using conscious strategies rather than simply using intuitive judgments or "rules of thumb." This phase is the most challenging segment of health information seeking and serves as a determinant of success (or lack thereof) in the information-seeking process. The following section on Sources of Health Information further explains this phase.

The fifth phase is *information management*, whereby one has to organize information that has been gathered in some manner to ensure easy retrieval and use in the future. The last phase is *information use*, in which one will synthesize information found across various resources, draw conclusions, and locate the answer to his or her original question and/or the content that fulfills the information need. This phase also often involves implementation, such as using the information to solve a health problem; make health-related decisions; identify and engage in behaviors that will help a person to avoid health risks; share the health information found with family members and friends who may benefit from it; and advocate more broadly for personal, family, or community health.

## The Importance of Health Literacy

The conception of health has moved from a passive view (someone is either well or ill) to one that is more active and process based (someone is working toward preventing or managing disease). Hence, the dominant focus has shifted from doctors and treatments to patients and prevention, resulting in the need to strengthen our ability and confidence (as patients and consumers of health care) to look for, assess, understand, manage, share, adapt, and use health-related information. An individual's health literacy level has been found to predict his or her health status better than age, race, educational attainment, employment status, and income level (National Network of Libraries of Medicine, 2013). Greater health literacy also enables individuals to better communicate with health care providers such as doctors, nutritionists, and therapists, as they can pose more relevant, informed, and useful questions to health care providers. Another added advantage of greater health literacy is better information-seeking skills, not only for health but also in other domains, such as completing assignments for school.

## Sources of Health Information: The Good, the Bad, and the In-Between

For generations, doctors, nurses, nutritionists, health coaches, and other health professionals have been the trusted sources of health information. Additionally, researchers have found that young adults, when they have health-related questions, typically turn to a family member who has had firsthand experience with a health condition because of their family member's close proximity and because of their past experience with, and trust in, this individual. Expertise should be a core consideration when consulting a person, website, or book for health information. The credentials and background of the person or author and conflicting interests of the author (and his or her organization) must be checked and validated to ensure the likely credibility of the health information they are conveying. While books often have implied credibility because of the peer-review process involved, self-publishing has challenged this credibility, so qualifications of book authors should also be verified. When it comes to health information, currency of the source must also be examined. When examining health information/studies presented, pay attention to the exhaustiveness of research methods utilized to offer recommendations or conclusions. Small and nondiverse sample size is often—but not always—an indication of reduced credibility. Studies that confuse correlation with causation are another potential issue to watch for. Information seekers must also pay attention to the sponsors of the research studies. For example, if a study is sponsored by manufacturers of drug Y and the study recommends that drug Y is the best treatment to manage or cure a disease, this may indicate a lack of objectivity on the part of the researchers.

The Internet is rapidly becoming one of the main sources of health information. Online forums, news agencies, personal blogs, social media sites, pharmacy sites, and celebrity "doctors" are all offering medical and health information targeted to various types of people in regard to all types of diseases and symptoms. There are professional journalists, citizen journalists, hoaxers, and people paid to write fake health news on various sites that may appear to have a legitimate domain name and may even have authors who claim to have professional credentials such as an MD. All these sites *may* offer useful information or information that appears to be useful and relevant; however, much of the information may be debatable and may fall into gray areas that require readers to discern credibility, reliability, and biases.

While broad recognition and acceptance of certain media, institutions, and people often serve as the most popular determining factors to assess credibility of health information among young people, keep in mind that there are legitimate Internet sites, databases, and books that publish health information and serve as sources of health information for doctors, other health sites, and members of the public. For example, MedlinePlus (https://medlineplus.gov) has trusted sources on over 975 diseases and conditions and presents the information in easy-to-understand language.

The chart here presents factors to consider when assessing credibility of health information. However, keep in mind that these factors function only as a guide and require continuous updating to keep abreast with the changes in the landscape of health information, information sources, and technologies.

The chart can serve as a guide; however, approaching a librarian about how one can go about assessing the credibility of both print and online health information is far more effective than using generic checklist-type tools. While librarians are not health experts, they can apply and teach patrons strategies to determine the credibility of health information.

With the prevalence of fake sites and fake resources that appear to be legitimate, it is important to use the following health information assessment tips to verify health information that one has obtained (St. Jean et al., 2015, p. 151):

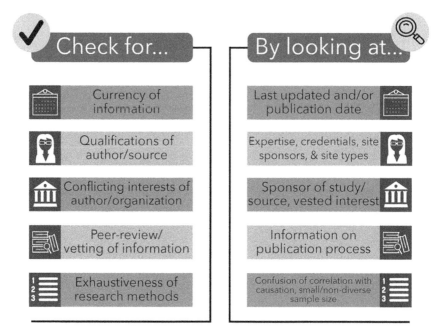

All images from flaticon.com

- **Don't assume you are right**: Even when you feel very sure about an answer, keep in mind that the answer may not be correct, and it is important to conduct (further) searches to validate the information.
- **Don't assume you are wrong**: You may actually have correct information, even if the information you encounter does not match—that is, you may be right and the resources that you have found may contain false information.
- **Take an open approach**: Maintain a critical stance by not including your preexisting beliefs as keywords (or letting them influence your choice of keywords) in a search, as this may influence what it is possible to find out.
- **Verify, verify, and verify**: Information found, especially on the Internet, needs to be validated, no matter how the information appears on the site (i.e., regardless of the appearance of the site or the quantity of information that is included).

Health literacy comes with experience navigating health information. Professional sources of health information, such as doctors, health care providers, and health databases, are still the best, but one also has the power to search for health information and then verify it by consulting with these trusted sources and by using the health information assessment tips and guide shared previously.

Mega Subramaniam, PhD

Associate Professor, College of Information Studies,

University of Maryland

## References and Further Reading

American Association of School Librarians (AASL). (2009). *Standards for the 21st-Century Learner in Action*. Chicago, IL: American Association of School Librarians.

Hilligoss, B., & Rieh, S. Y. (2008). Developing a unifying framework of credibility assessment: Construct, heuristics, and interaction in context. *Information Processing & Management*, 44(4), 1467–84.

Kuhlthau, C. C. (1988). Developing a model of the library search process: Cognitive and affective aspects. *Reference Quarterly*, 28(2), 232–42.

National Network of Libraries of Medicine (NNLM). (2013). Health literacy. Bethesda, MD: National Network of Libraries of Medicine. Retrieved from nnlm.gov/outreach/consumer/hlthlit.html

Ratzan, S. C., & Parker, R. M. (2000). Introduction. In C. R. Selden, M. Zorn, S. C. Ratzan, & R. M. Parker (Eds.), *National Library of Medicine current bibliographies in medicine: Health literacy*. NLM Pub. No. CBM 2000–1. Bethesda, MD: National Institutes of Health, U.S. Department of Health and Human Services.

St. Jean, B., Taylor, N. G., Kodama, C., & Subramaniam, M. (February 2017). Assessing the health information source perceptions of tweens using card-sorting exercises. *Journal of Information Science*. Retrieved from http://journals.sagepub.com/doi/abs/10.1177/0165551516687728

St. Jean, B., Subramaniam, M., Taylor, N. G., Follman, R., Kodama, C., & Casciotti, D. (2015). The influence of positive hypothesis testing on youths' online health-related information seeking. *New Library World*, 116(3/4), 136–54.

Subramaniam, M., St. Jean, B., Taylor, N. G., Kodama, C., Follman, R., & Casciotti, D. (2015). Bit by bit: Using design-based research to improve the health literacy of adolescents. *JMIR Research Protocols*, 4(2), paper e62. Retrieved from http://www.ncbi.nlm.nih.gov/pmc/articles/PMC4464334/

Valenza, J. (2016, November 26). Truth, truthiness, and triangulation: A news literacy toolkit for a "post-truth" world [Web log]. Retrieved from http://blogs.slj.com/neverendingsearch/2016/11/26/truth-truthiness-triangulation-and-the-librarian-way-a-news-literacy-toolkit-for-a-post-truth-world/

# Common Misconceptions about Epidemics and Pandemics

## 1. Epidemics are caused by highly communicable microbial agents

Epidemics are caused by communicable disease, but they need not be highly communicable. Diseases like tuberculosis and HIV/AIDS are not highly communicable and yet have been some of the most significant and lethal epidemics of the twenty-first century. Tuberculosis can take as long as ten weeks from the time of exposure before infection occurs. The time from exposure to infection with AIDS can be anywhere from one to fifteen years or longer. Indeed, communicable diseases with long incubation periods tend to get less public attention because they don't trigger our fight or flight instincts. For more information, see questions 7, 9, and 10.

## 2. Epidemics are only caused by novel pathogens for which humans have no immunity

There are hundreds of pathogens with which humans have been living with for thousands of years without immunity. Diseases like cholera, typhoid, influenza, plague, and tuberculosis are not novel diseases yet have caused millions of deaths in the last 100 years. More importantly, very few Americans have been vaccinated for cholera, tuberculosis, typhoid, or plague. Even when vaccines are available the supply may be inadequate in the event of an outbreak. Epidemics continue to emerge from diseases where insufficient efforts have been made to improve immunity from reliable and safe vaccines. For more information, see questions 3 and 11.

## 3. Pandemics are the result of the highly interconnected world we live in, where no country is more than 24 hours away from any other

Not all disease requires close contact or short incubation periods to spread around the world. The speed at which a pathogen may be transmitted is only one factor that influences the potential for a pandemic scale disease. Diseases like tuberculosis and HIV/AIDS may take years to spread across the world—simply because they are less transmissible and have longer incubation periods. Moreover, in the case of zoonotic diseases like avian flu, transmission is not related to the interconnected world of humans. It reflects the highly mobile world of wild birds travelling across continents and infecting chickens that in turn infect farmers. Farm workers then become the vehicles for transmitting the disease to the rest of humanity. For more information, see questions 7 and 9.

## 4. Epidemics are only dangerous for people who are already unhealthy

This is a common misconception for those who believe their robust health is enough to shield them from disease. Diseases like yellow fever, malaria, and Zika are vector-borne diseases transmitted by mosquitoes and can infect anyone of any age, or state of health. They infect everyone who is bitten by a mosquito carrying the pathogens causing these diseases. Being healthy doesn't stop you from getting disease or guarantee you won't get a serious case. It also doesn't preclude you from experiencing many other hardships such as an inability to work, attend school, obtain health care or avoid depression or other mental health issues. Yet getting infected may be less severe for those with a strong immune system. Similarly, anyone receiving an infectious dose of the pathogens causing Ebola, cholera, and typhoid will succumb to disease but recovery favors those in the best of health. The infectious dose is influenced by the immune competence of each individual. For more information, see questions 38 and 40.

## 5. More investment in vaccine research and development can prevent future epidemics

This is an unrealistic dream based on the hope we can develop vaccines for all known diseases, future variants of disease and novel pathogens that have not yet been identified. Preventing disease means achieving a high level of vaccination across the world for all known communicable disease. This is simply beyond the resources available in the world today. Avoiding future pandemics through vaccine research and development is a laudable but financially impractical goal. A case in point are novel pathogens. How can vaccines prevent pandemics caused by novel pathogens? Novel diseases are being discovered on an annual basis. Those making vaccine investments would be hard pressed to identify and prioritize research objectives without any knowledge of the lethality, transmissibility, or pathogen reservoirs of any given pathogen. Novel pathogens are the trump card that ensures vaccines will never prevent epidemics. At best they will be an important response to an epidemic caused by a novel pathogen. For more information see questions 2, 6, 7, and 15.

# Questions and Answers

# The Basics

## 1. What is an epidemic? What is a pandemic?

There are numerous definitions of an epidemic reflecting varying interests of individuals and organizations using this term. The term "epidemic" has historically referred to communicable disease normally absent in any given population but appears for the first time, or after many years since its previous appearance, and spreads relatively rapidly often with severe outcomes for human health. Epidemics appear with a frequency clearly in excess of past expectations. An epidemic exists when the following criteria are met: (1) there is rapid increase in the number of cases, (2) the infectious agent is easily transmitted, (3) the exposed population is large or the pathogen adversely targets vulnerable populations, (4) there is little or no immunity to the disease, and (5) the time and place of the outbreak is unprecedented.

These criteria are intended as guides used by county public health officers and state public health directors, in evaluating the evidence at hand, when deciding if epidemic conditions exist. For example, a single case of a communicable disease long absent from a population or the first invasion by a disease not previously recognized in a region requires immediate reporting and a full epidemiological investigation. According to the American Public Health Association (APHA), two cases of such a disease associated in time and place are enough evidence of transmission to be considered an epidemic. The APHA's emphasis on the critical role of surveillance of the initial cases is intended to focus efforts on a proactive approach to the control of epidemics—not on speculating about the possible speed at which the disease might spread.

At the time of the initial discovery of a case of communicable disease, public health officials refer to the person as "patient zero." If more cases are identified then, these are referred to as a cluster and if the disease spreads the term "outbreak" is used. Surveillance and public health measures determine if an outbreak becomes an epidemic. It is critical to identify a communicable disease in the population as early as possible so a rapid public health intervention can hopefully stop a potential epidemic in its tracks. Should those efforts fail, and the disease spreads beyond one municipality or county, then an epidemic condition may be declared. This stepwise approach avoids overreacting to a few cases of disease and declaring an epidemic before public health interventions have had time to work.

In contrast to the APHA's definition of an epidemic, the World Health Organization (WHO) uses four criteria to determine if epidemic conditions exist. Instead of using the term "outbreak," the WHO uses the term "event" and defines it as "a manifestation of disease or an occurrence that creates a potential for disease." For an event to become an epidemic it must have (1) a public health impact, including (2) a significant risk of international spread, (3) be unusual or unexpected, and (4) merit international restrictions. If two or more of these conditions exist, WHO can declare an epidemic exists.

A pandemic is an epidemic encompassing a wide geographic area involving multiple nations and spreading in an exponential way—where the number of cases of disease is far more than those previously reported. Pandemics are called "a public health emergency of international concern" (PHEIC). A PHEIC need not be a communicable disease and for this reason the primary determinant of whether an epidemic exists is (1) if an "event" meets two of the four WHO criteria set forth in the International Health Regulations or if it is one of four specific diseases (smallpox, wild type poliomyelitis, SARS, or any new subtype of human influenza). These four diseases automatically trigger a PHEIC without requiring the four-tier test mentioned above.

The mere act of labelling any disease as a pandemic has enormous social, economic, and political implications. When the WHO declares the existence of a pandemic, this decision triggers nations to commit significant financial and human resources to respond to the anticipated threat—a challenge when limited fiscal resources exist. Yet despite these economic, social, and political concerns associated with declaring a "public health emergency of international concern," it is through declarations of an impending worst-case public health crisis that nations activate rapid response measures. When implemented at the earliest stage of an outbreak such measures have a much greater ability to influence the spread of disease than those implemented months later. Rapid response measures may not stop a pandemic in its tracks—but may at least slow its spread. Epidemic diseases may become pandemics if public health countermeasures are not successful.

During the last seventy years, the term "epidemic" has also been used by epidemiologists in an informal way to identify the prevalence of certain patterns of behavior or phenomena such as an epidemic of obesity or an epidemic of violence. These definitions are not infectious disease epidemics. However, the field of epidemiology has largely ignored classic definitions of an epidemic and applied the term to phenomena of a non-infectious nature. It should be pointed out outbreaks of communicable disease may often not be fully understood until years later when its mode of transmission is better understood than at the time of an outbreak. In some cases, it has taken years to determine the mode of transmission or even if a disease is communicable. For example, in the nineteenth century, Pellagra—a disease caused by a lack of niacin (one of the components of a vitamin B complex)—was thought to be communicable due to its widespread presence in prison populations in several southern states. After the US Public Health Service examined the prisoner's diet and altered their daily menu the disease disappeared. The principles of epidemiology in this context were indispensable in determining the causative factors of disease and its non-infectious nature. The disease had taken hold within the prison population, but its cause was a diet composed of meat, meal—cornmeal—and molasses which did not provide the vitamin B complex. Epidemiology in this instance determined the disease was not a communicable disease epidemic but a dietary deficiency.

At the opposite extreme tuberculosis was not considered a communicable disease in nineteenth-century America. Lacking an understanding of its communicability until the early twentieth-century American physicians failed to apply appropriate public health measures consistent with its contagious character. TB was the most lethal communicable disease in nineteenth-century America yet despite being an epidemic it was thought to be an inherited disease analogous to a genetic disorder. For this reason, nineteenth-century public health officials never declared TB to be an epidemic. Another more recent example of a misclassified disease is vaginal cancer—a communicable disease formerly classified by its outcome—cancer. Vaginal cancer is caused by the human papillomavirus, a pathogen that infects an estimated 570,000 new cases annually. Indeed, about 5 percent of cancers are attributable to HPV.

While the field of epidemiology originated from the study of infectious disease in human populations, epidemiologists now study a wide range of diseases and public health concerns to determine causes, modes of transmission and impacted populations. Based on the range of errors made in the past, it is only appropriate for epidemiologists to investigate all forms of disease regardless of their presumed communicability or lack thereof. For novel disease, the cause of illness is not always immediately apparent and for this reason the expansion of the field of epidemiology to address a broad range of disease and public health conditions may often identify diseases that have been misclassified with respect to their causative factors.

Public health officers need to understand the mode of transmission, its communicability, the potential exposure of people with little or no immunity to the disease and the availability of public health interventions before declaring a communicable disease outbreak. If the outbreak cannot be controlled and spreads rapidly, an epidemic exists. In turn, if the epidemic spreads to multiple nations the WHO may declare a PHEIC indicating a pandemic exists.

## 2.  Which diseases are most likely to cause epidemics and pandemics?

The most likely diseases to cause epidemics are those most easily transmitted—whether that be by drinking contaminated water (e.g., cholera), inhaling bacteria or viruses (e.g., pneumonic plague, tuberculosis, measles, Severe Acute Respiratory Symptom) or through vectors such as mosquitoes that carry dengue, malaria, yellow fever, or Zika. Many of these diseases are commonly found in areas where it is difficult to control mosquitoes or where public water supplies do not exist or have been compromised by leaking pipes or poor sanitary measures. Vector-borne disease already exists in many parts of the world including North and South America, Africa, and many Asian nations where public health measures have failed to control their spread.

A second category of disease that could cause an epidemic or even a pandemic are novel pathogens—those that previously did not infect humans. A novel pathogen may be one that infects species with similar genetic characteristics to humans, rodents, mammals, and primates. Diseases transmitted from animals to humans are called zoonotic diseases. They represent a significant source for lethal pathogens that could trigger a future epidemic. For example, it is believed fruit bats are the reservoir for filoviridae, the viral pathogen causing Ebola. For many years, Ebola was a disease of nonhuman primates, limited to its geographic range within several remote locations in Africa. However, human exposure to Ebola began to occur when people came into close contact with primates including eating these animals to supplement their diet. Since Ebola is transmitted by contact, this disease spread rapidly in African nations where cultural practices included touching the dead. Touching the dead body before burial created a mode of exposure with serious public health consequences. Diseases transmitted through contact with infected animals or people can infect many others quite rapidly unless public health measures are instituted to stop inappropriate behavior. For many years, it was not clear how

Ebola was transmitted to humans. Lack of knowledge increased the range of public health efforts used to tighten controls on human exposure—an effort that sometimes backfired when families felt their rights were being infringed. Control of epidemics requires an understanding of the mode by which infection is transmitted. Without this basic understanding overly controlling public health measures can be counter-productive, worsening the epidemic. Public understanding of how disease is transmitted plays a critical role in influencing human behavior and improving public health.

A third category of epidemics are those caused by mutations of known bacteria or viruses over time. An existing pathogen—whether a virus or a bacterium—may acquire genetic features making it capable of infecting humans more effectively than it had before. A mutation could make a pathogen more lethal or more communicable than it was before (see question 15). Overuse of antibiotics or antivirals may contribute to an acceleration of this natural process—especially when medicines are not properly taken as prescribed. Antibiotics that fail to eliminate bacteria from the body have the effect of selectively improving those that survive. The result of misused or overused antibiotics leads to antibiotic resistant strains and this has already happened in the case of *Mycobacterium tuberculosis* (the bacterium causing tuberculosis) and *Staphylococcus aureus*. Lacking effective antibiotic treatments these two diseases represent a clear and present danger; they could trigger epidemics without modern medicines to prevent infection.

Similarly, a number of viral diseases, such as pandemic influenza or possible future variants of Covid-19, are likely to pose the greatest threat. They are both hard to control through vaccines. Covid-19 is a special concern. It is not only easily transmitted by infected individuals, but asymptomatic individuals can also infect others as well. Pandemic influenza and future variants of Covid-19 are regarded as some of the greatest threats to humanity. Both mutate rapidly over short periods of time making it far more difficult to stockpile effective vaccines.

## 3. Are there places on earth where epidemic diseases are more common?

Three factors influence the geographic areas where epidemic disease is most common: (1) the proximity and frequency of human exposure to domestic or wild animals when the latter serve as reservoirs for disease; (2) the lack of sanitary conditions with respect to public water supplies in many parts of the world—increasing the chances of spreading waterborne diseases like cholera; and (3) the prevalence of vectors that transmit disease especially mosquito-borne disease.

The destruction of forests throughout the world is a contributing factor to the emergence of epidemic disease—especially those originating from novel pathogens. In some cases, tropical forests are being converted into farmland or cash crops such as palm tree oil, coffee, or even poppy production. The loss of forests eliminates the ecosystem upon which many species depend for their survival. It also brings these species into closer contact with humans—increasing the probability novel zoonotic pathogens unique to a small region find homes throughout the world. Over the last fifty years humans have been brought into closer contact with pathogens that had little or no contact with the world at large. Ebola is an example of a disease that was limited to nations in Central Africa including the Democratic Republic of Congo, Ghana, Guinea, Nigeria, Sierra Leone, Senegal, Sudan, and Uganda. In 2014, it spread to the United States and this triggered intense public concern on its potential to become an American epidemic.

Vector-borne disease such as malaria, dengue, yellow fever, and Zika are still quite common in tropical parts of the world. These diseases are found in parts of Southeast Asia, the sub-Saharan region of Africa and the heavily forested regions of South America including Brazil and Venezuela. Yellow fever is also found in the sub-Saharan regions of Africa including Congo, Sudan, and Uganda and in South America within Bolivia, Brazil, Colombia, Peru, and Venezuela. Dengue is found throughout South America, Africa, and Asia with an estimated 50 to 100 million infections annually. Zika infects as many as 1 million people annually. Latin America and the Caribbean are the primary locations where Zika outbreaks have occurred in recent years.

Another factor facilitating epidemic scale disease is when population growth outstrips the resources available to meet sustainable standards of living. Often this means a lack of access to sanitary sources of food and water and a poor or non-existent health care system to combat epidemic disease. Epidemics are more frequent when people are forced to live together in very close contact under less than adequate living conditions. Mass migrations of people caused by war, famine, or pestilence have been major causes of epidemic disease in the twentieth and twenty-first centuries. Humanitarian refugee camps in countries like Afghanistan, Bangladesh, Biafra, Ethiopia, Indonesia, Lebanon, Pakistan, Philippines, Syria, and Turkey have been reservoirs for epidemic disease. These refugee camps are beset with filth related disease such as cholera, and typhus and disease associated with crowding such as tuberculosis. Poor health, malnutrition, and the stresses of living in sub-standard living arrangements increase the chances refugees will be more vulnerable to epidemic disease.

Millions of people in this world struggle to make a living with no reliable source of food or water and limited resources to improve their lot. Lack of education, particularly when it is not equitably provided to both men and women, can adversely influence their personal health. For example, in countries where public education is provided, students have a better chance of learning skills to make better choices in life including personal hygiene and health practices. Education is a great antidote to many forms of disease—especially waterborne and foodborne diseases. Adopting practices such as boiling or purifying water and cooking raw foods are examples of the benefits of a basic public health education. Lack of education for women is an issue in Afghanistan and several African nations where women are not encouraged to attend school. Indeed, they may be prohibited from doing so.

Epidemic disease can also be found in the wet markets of China where live animals are sold for food and this practice creates an easy pathway for the spread of zoonotic disease to humans. Viral disease like SARS or Covid-19 have been identified as caused by viral discharges of infected animals to which humans are exposed. This same process also occurs at poultry farms in the Midwestern United States when wild geese infected with an avian flu encounter domesticated chickens or ducks that in turn come into close contact with humans. Wherever humans have close and sustained exposure to mammals, and to a lesser extend with birds, serving as carriers of flu like illnesses these places serve as incubators of disease.

## 4. Who decides when an epidemic has emerged and who decides when it's over? What criteria are used to do so?

In the United States, state governors are responsible for deciding when an epidemic has emerged based on the recommendations of state or county public health officials. That decision is based on at least three factors; first, whether the disease is considered communicable through human-to-human transmission or through vector-borne transmission. Secondly, governors must consider the rate at which the disease multiplies based on the best available evidence from reported cases of the disease. Finally, the decision must consider the likelihood public health countermeasures such as vaccines, quarantine, isolation, or vector controls can be implemented quickly. If these measures fail to stop the spread of the disease from its first reported case within a short period of time public health authorities will declare an outbreak has occurred. Declaring the existence of an "epidemic" raises public concerns—including panic and, in some cases, an urge to flee the area where the outbreak exists. For these reasons, public health officials use the word "outbreak" to describe the initial discovery of a communicable disease.

Epidemics may last a few weeks to several years depending upon the public health countermeasures taken, the communicability of the disease and the herd immunity of the population. Herd immunity occurs when people either have survived exposure to a disease or have achieved immunity through a vaccine. The greater the number of people who are immune to a disease the less able the pathogen can infect other people. Herd immunity is a key concept influencing the length of time an epidemic persists. Some highly communicable diseases like measles require nearly 95 percent of the population to be immunized before the epidemic subsides. Vaccines provide an important means of stopping epidemics. They are especially useful for those never exposed to a disease or whose immunity has waned due to the passage of time since their last vaccination.

As the immunity of a population increases the community level susceptibility to that disease declines. Epidemics decline when the basic reproductive number for the disease is smaller than its ability to maintain its growth. One way to understand this concept is by applying the basic reproductive number to human population growth. For example, if a hypothetical family has three children and each of the three children gets married and they each have three children, and their children in turn get married and have three children, the basic reproductive number for that family's growth is three (3). However, if that same father and mother only have one child and their child marries but decides not to have children the basic reproductive number for that family would be in decline—going from 1 to 0.5 to 0. When this happens, the population is in decline. Moreover, if there are no progeny amongst all these successive families and their progeny the population will disappear. Similarly, the same basic reproductive number principle applies to the spread or decline of disease.

Depending on the disease's rate of decline, public health officials may declare the epidemic or pandemic over. A disease need not be eliminated for a state governor to declare, based on advice from the health commissioner and other department heads, an epidemic over. As long as the basic reproductive number— as measured by the cases of the disease—declines and public health measures are influencing that decline, then the epidemic can be declared over. That decision is never based on the complete elimination of the disease. It also must consider the ability to control isolated hot spots, and with due consideration of the adverse consequences the epidemic or pandemic has on the economy and the social life of the people. If public health were only measured by the elimination of an epidemic disease, there would be many unintended consequences. For example, hundreds of thousands were unable to work or visit family and friends during extended lockdowns, curfews, school closings, and other public health measures during Covid-19. Lockdowns adversely affect the ability of people to make a living and maintain a healthy state of mind. Declaring an epidemic or pandemic over can never be made without considering the long-term economic and social consequences of isolation on people and their livelihood.

## 5. What have been the most lethal epidemics in recorded history?

The most lethal epidemics in human history have been caused by smallpox, bubonic plague, cholera, yellow fever, and pandemic influenza. Since there are different ways of defining what constitutes a lethal epidemic, let's review some of the ways past epidemics have been declared lethal. The lethality of an epidemic can be measured by its case fatality rate—the number of people who died after exposure to the disease. This approach has only been useful in the modern era where public health agencies have tracked the number of cases of illness as well as the number of deaths. Since those measurements were rarely kept in earlier periods in history, the second method of estimating the lethality of a disease is by the total number of deaths or the percentage of the entire population that died from a disease. Even these measurements are often mere estimates or wild guesses when cities or nations fail to maintain a census of their population and/ or do not track the causes of death. Yet despite these challenges, making death estimates are inevitable even in the modern era since not all disease or deaths are reported or, when reported, may be improperly categorized to avoid stigmatizing the individuals who died from a horrid and socially repugnant infection.

Over the last two millennia hundreds of millions of people died from smallpox. With a case fatality rate as high as 30 percent, it was also one of the most feared diseases because it scarred its victims with raw oozing pustules often covering the entire body including the inner airways and other exposure points. Those who survived were often permanently scarred and many were blinded for life. Smallpox struck in the Roman era resulting in an estimated 3.5 to 7 million deaths during the years 164 to 165 AD. This was one of the worst epidemics during the Roman Empire (Donald Hopkins, 1983). Similar waves of smallpox appeared throughout Europe and Asia up until the twentieth century. Dozens of books have been written about the catastrophic impacts of smallpox on eastern and western cultures. It was especially prevalent in regions of the world that maintained trading partnerships with Europeans. North and South America remained free of smallpox until the arrival of the Spanish Conquistadors in Mexico and the French and English in North America. After their arrival, as many as 90 percent of Native Americans lost their lives to smallpox during the sixteenth and seventeenth centuries. They had no natural immunity to the disease.

Similarly bubonic plague—a form of disease transmitted by the rat flea to humans—is also extremely lethal. If the symptoms of plague are not identified early and an antibiotic taken within days of exposure the chances of death are high. The plague, a disease caused by the bacterium *Yersinia pestis,* can sometimes be transmitted in its pneumonic form by exhalations of those infected. Pneumonic plague has an incubation period of one to four days and without treatment the chances of death are extremely high.

The plague struck Europe during three major waves over the last 1,500 years. The first major epidemic occurred in the sixth century and was known as the Justinian Plague killing an estimated 3 to 7 million people. The second major plague epidemic, known as the Black Plague of the fourteenth century, killed an estimated 75 million people or 35 percent of the entire population of Europe. It is considered the single worst epidemic in recorded history. Smaller epidemics of bubonic plague struck England in the sixteenth and seventeenth centuries including the most famous great plague of 1665 that resulted in an enormous loss of life in the greater London area. An estimated 100,000 of the 460,000 people in the greater London area died in the 1665 epidemic, or about 22 percent of the entire population. The third wave of the plague occurred in the period 1894 to 1912 impacting Asia, Africa, and even the United States. An estimated 13 million died of the plague during this period.

The Spanish flu was the most lethal pandemic of the twentieth century. The death rate was exacerbated by the First World War and the concentration of soldiers in tight quarters in barracks, on transport ships, and on the battlefield. One way to understand the lethality of the world's first modern pandemic is to compare the loss of life from the Spanish flu to the First World War battlefield casualties. An estimated 16 million people lost their lives on the battlefield or from the unintended consequences of that war. In contrast, an estimated 50 million people died from the Spanish flu during the period 1917 to 1919. At that time, the medical authorities had no idea what caused this disease and no vaccines existed to prevent it.

The Covid-19 pandemic of 2020 to 2023 is the most lethal pandemic of the twenty-first century with over 5 million reported lives lost on a worldwide basis. However, because of the limited reporting of cases in many nations of the world, the WHO estimates an additional 14.3 million excess deaths are attributable to Covid-19. Despite the end of state and federal-level emergency public health measures throughout the United States, Covid-19 continues to infect thousands of people on a daily basis. Unlike the Spanish flu, medical scientists were able to develop vaccines to prevent or, at least reduce the severity of Covid-19. Remarkably, Covid-19 vaccines were released under an Emergency Use Authorization within less than twelve months of the onset of the pandemic. The approval of multiple vaccines by the Food and Drug Administration and the Centers for Disease Control and Prevention represents an historic leap forward in our timely ability to respond to viral pathogens. Yet despite the development of several vaccine options, many people died prior to their availability. Furthermore, many died simply because they failed to get vaccinated—either through vaccine hesitancy or due to less than optimum public health education measures concerning the benefits of vaccination.

Cholera was one of the most lethal of the nineteenth-century diseases affecting Europe and the Western Hemisphere. Its causative agent *Vibrio cholerae* creates profuse watery stools resulting in a massive loss of body water and its electrolytes and leads to dehydration and often death for half of those infected—unless treated. There were at least four waves of cholera that struck the United States starting in 1832, 1849, 1866, and 1892. Cases of cholera predominantly arrived in eastern port cities through the arrival of infected immigrants. Medical historian Charles Rosenberg called cholera the classic epidemic disease of the nineteenth century. It was one of the most common and lethal of the diseases to strike American port cities and, until Robert Koch's discovery of the *Vibrio cholerae* bacterium in 1884, the medical profession only knew it was transmitted by contaminated water but had no idea what pathogen was responsible for infecting humans. While no accurate tally exists of all those who died from this disease in the nineteenth century, tens of thousands lost their lives during these four epidemic waves.

Yellow fever struck east coast port cities of the United States during the late eighteenth century and even throughout much of the nineteenth century. It was especially prevalent in southern port cities, like New Orleans, where a warmer climate played an important role in its survival. Yellow fever is a mosquito-borne disease carried by *Aedes aegypti*. These mosquitos thrive in warm weather a fact that turns out to be an important prerequisite for determining where it poses the greatest threat to human health. Fortunately, cold weather, especially two consecutive hours with temperatures below freezing will kill *Aedes aegypti*.

While yellow fever is a warm weather threat, protective measures depend on understanding its cause and lethality. With a short incubation period of three to six days, yellow fever infection is a serious concern. Those infected have a case fatality rate from 2 to 12 percent. Moreover, there is no antiviral treatment for those not vaccinated. Yellow fever remains a lethal disease in the tropical regions of the world.

While we now know yellow fever is a vector-borne disease, in the nineteenth century no one understood it was transmitted by mosquitoes. Instead, the prevalent beliefs were it (1) was caused either by foul air associated with putrescible wastes, sewer gases, or other rotting matter or by (2) a lack of sanitation especially on-board ships. Some physicians noticed yellow fever was associated with the arrival of ships from the tropics during the summer months. Poor on board sanitation was blamed for numerous yellow fever epidemics. Tens of thousands of American died from yellow fever during the period 1790 to 1803. Furthermore, in one three-month period in the summer of 1853 a total of 6,442 residents of New Orleans died from yellow fever. Almost twenty-five years later, in 1878, yellow fever returned with a vengeance in the southern states infecting 120,000 people. As many as 20,000 died—making it the most lethal yellow fever epidemic in American history.

Perhaps the most forgotten of all epidemics is that of tuberculosis. It was the most lethal communicable disease found in nineteenth-century America. In 1880, when the US Census investigated the causes of death in America it determined consumption was responsible for 91,270 deaths in that year. Undoubtedly, based on this one-year nationwide study, millions died from tuberculosis in the nineteenth century. This was the greatest cause of death in America in 1880 and also during the previous thirty years (US Census Report on the Mortality and Vital Statistics of the United States, 1880). For virtually the entire nineteenth century tuberculosis—also called consumption in that era—was not understood to be a communicable disease. Indeed, even after 1882 when Robert Koch determined the disease was caused by the highly contagious bacterium *Mycobacterium tuberculosis*, American physicians still did not consider it communicable. In contrast, European physicians knew it to be so.

It was not until the beginning of the First World War that most American states declared it a communicable disease. The result of the long delay in educating the public and the medical profession of its contagious and highly lethal nature, meant millions of Americans died. These deaths reflected an absence of appropriate preventive measures to stop its spread. Tuberculosis is an example of a highly communicable disease that was misdiagnosed as an inherited illness that spread in what might be called an epidemic of ignorance.

## 6. Does climate change influence the prevalence of epidemic disease?

Climate change has been demonstrated to influence the geographic range of many vector-borne diseases. There are three ways climate change effects the prevalence of communicable disease: (1) higher temperatures have expanded the geographic range and stimulated the proliferation and reproductive rates of vector-borne disease; (2) more intense floods have led to increases in vector and waterborne disease; and (3) more intense droughts have led to mass migrations of millions of people and this in turn has created unhealthy living conditions, inadequate diets, and weakened immunity to vector and waterborne disease.

For example, *Yersinia pestis*, the bacterium that causes bubonic plague, is found throughout southwestern United States. Its original entry into San Francisco Bay took place on a vessel coming from China in the year 1900. After arriving in the San Francisco Bay area rats carried the plague throughout California and into southwestern United States. The rat fleas eventually infected ground squirrels, rabbits, and other rodents by transmitting the *Yersinia pestis* pathogen through its bite. As the climate gets warmer, ground squirrels and other rodents of the southwest can be expected to move northward into Canada and higher elevations. In addition, recent studies have already demonstrated increases in the population of fleas in the southwest due to higher temperatures. Since fleas are responsible for up to 70 percent of the plague transmitted in the southwestern United States, their increased population is expected to increase the potential for bubonic plague to become more severe. Climate change is not only expanding the geographic range of the plague it increases the potential for more severe outbreaks throughout the southwestern states.

A warming climate has also changed the geographic range of disease carrying mosquitoes in South America leading to a 31 percent increase in the number of months suitable for malaria transmission further up South American mountain sides previously too cold and dry to support their survival. Similarly, a study sponsored by the 2021 Lancet Countdown Report found a 39 percent increase in the number of months suitable for malaria transmission in highland areas of the world. These findings have been corroborated by the Intergovernmental Panel on Climate Change (IPCC) Sixth Assessment Report. The IPCC confirms a warming climate will have the greatest impact on malaria cases in Africa. Indeed, Africa has the greatest burden of malaria with more than 90 percent of world-wide malaria deaths found on that continent.

A warming climate is expanding the zones in which cholera can survive including several high latitude areas of the world (e.g., the Baltics, the Pacific Northwest, and the Atlantic Northeast). Similarly, Bangladesh has experienced an increasing presence of cholera coinciding with El Niño Southern Oscillations (ENSO) that increase temperatures, compared to earlier periods in Bangladesh history where these oscillations were not as pronounced. El Niño is the name given to the warming of the Pacific Ocean that occurs on an irregular basis and can affect weather patterns throughout the world. Rising sea surface temperatures attributable to El Niño also influence the marine ecology of the Bangladesh coast that in turn increases the prevalence of human cholera which poses a health hazard varying with the seasonal warming of the sea.

Another way a changing climate influences the spread of disease is by dislocation effects created by droughts, floods, hurricanes, and extreme weather events. The duration and severity of droughts and floods have regularly triggered mass migrations of people seeking refuge. Droughts are the precursor to famines and these in turn often trigger mass migrations leading to potentially serious outbreaks of disease. For example, when entire populations suffer from a lack of food and water their immune systems weaken. Conditions are made even worse when people are concentrated in refugee camps with limited sanitary facilities—a perfect recipe for so-called filth-based diseases such as cholera and typhoid to take hold.

Mass migration induced by climate change is another consequence of mixing populations. Concentrating large numbers of people together also increases the potential for disease transmission from the migrant's home country to the country serving as the host for the refugees. Different immunity levels between the two populations as well as the existence of asymptomatic infections in one or both populations can lead to an inadvertent triggering of epidemic disease for which one or both populations have no immunity.

Efforts to support the humanitarian needs of hundreds of thousands of people seeking refuge are always well intended but often underfunded. Despite best efforts, humanitarian interventions are often unable to simultaneously overcome insufficient shelter, sanitary facilities, and food to meet the needs of tens of thousands of people. These conditions enable waterborne and contact-based diseases to spread.

It is important to recognize climate change is not the only factor improving the odds for more frequent epidemic scale disease. Often such factors as expanded systems of transportation, expanded international commerce and mass migrations between cultures, previously relatively isolated, work in tandem with a changing climate to accelerate pathogen transmission. In many cases it is difficult to tease out the unique contribution of a changing climate to the spread of disease. However, the study of the prevalence of cholera in Bangladesh is an example of a robust analysis of the direct link between that disease and more intense temperatures caused by the intensifying effects of the El Niño Southern Oscillation in a warming climate.

The 2022 IPCC has investigated the strength of the climate change impact on epidemic disease and concluded, with a high degree of confidence, epidemics of malaria, dengue, and other vector-borne diseases are expanding their habitats with a warming climate. The IPCC has also confirmed the scientific evidence supporting the growing threat of a warming climate on the dispersion of cholera in Bangladesh and Africa and in refugee camps. Similarly, the expanded prevalence of bubonic plague in the southwest United States is directly influenced by rising temperatures. The longer-term effects of climate change on human health are a topic of intense and ongoing research throughout the world. We can expect the links between communicable disease and climate change to evolve as we learn more about the changing migratory patterns of species, other than humans, and what consequences these migrations have on the transmission of disease.

## 7. Which diseases pose the greatest threat to humanity?

Diseases that pose the greatest threat to humanity are viral pathogens such as variants of Covid-19 and other pathogens easily transmitted in an aerosol form. Viral pathogens are capable of rapidly mutating thereby compromising the long-term effectiveness of vaccines. Since highly communicable disease pose a threat to large numbers of people, measles must also be considered a disease of international concern. As the most communicable disease in the world, measles, under certain conditions, can have a case fatality rate between 10 and 30 percent when vaccinations are not available and in locations such as refugee camps, communities with serious chronic undernutrition and in communities with poor access to public health services. While measles case fatality rates for developed nations are as low as 0.1 percent, let's not forget there are millions of people in third world nations who have neither the health, shelter, medical services, immunity, social support services, nor sanitary conditions to survive a more infectious measles variant. Perhaps more importantly, when we consider not only a potential natural mutation, but a bioengineered variant created by a rogue scientist, measles is a pathogen to place on the epidemic watch list. Any mutations that might alter the pathogenicity of measles in these circumstances is of great public health concern.

The mutagenicity of human pathogens is not a hypothetical question. During the years following the anthrax crisis, dozens of American scientists identified the most lethal pathogens with the express purpose of developing suitable public health countermeasures. As a result of the use of anthrax as a bioweapon against federal government facilities and news media outlets in 2001, the US Department of Health and Human Services promptly convened a group of scientists to identify pathogens and toxins that pose the greatest potential for mass casualties. That effort identified fifteen pathogens including Avian Influenza virus, Ebola and Marburg viruses, *Yersinia pestis* (the causative agent of the plague), Variola major virus (the causative agent of smallpox that now only exists in two top security biosafety laboratories in the world), and *Bacillus anthracis* (the causative agent of anthrax). These six select agents, a subset of the federal government's list of fifteen select agents, pose the greatest potential threat to humanity. These pathogens share three characteristics that make them dangerous: (1) their ease of transmission to humans, (2) the short incubation period between exposure and infection, and (3) their high fatality rate.

Unlike any other period in recorded history, scientists in the modern era have the ability to bioengineer more lethal and communicable forms of pathogens than already exist in nature. Research concerning the genetic characteristics of highly lethal pathogens has been authorized under strict controls by the US Department of Health and Human Services. However, such controls do not necessarily exist throughout the world. Controls over the development of biological weapons are governed under the Biological Weapons Convention of 1975, signed by 186 of the world's 196 nations. However, ten nation-states have not signed this treaty including Israel, Namibia, and South Sudan. Bad actors living in these states are not subject to government sanctions and therefore these states could serve as training grounds for bioterrorists seeking to turn microbial pathogens into weapons of war.

Surprising as it may seem, the Biological Weapons Convention does not prohibit the signatory nations from stockpiling lethal pathogens and for this reason the effectiveness of the convention depends upon the degree to which each nation maintains robust security controls over their existing stockpiles. America's experience with the release of anthrax spores from a government research laboratory in 2001 led to the closure of dozens of federal government and privately owned buildings in Washington, DC, and across the nation resulting from the receipt of anthrax laced letters in the mail. This example clearly reveals it takes more than merely signing a biological weapons convention to ensure weapons of mass destruction do not get misused. The risk of release of highly lethal pathogens from biosafety laboratories is not zero when there are thousands of actors with the skills to synthesize novel disease for which we have no immunity.

Another aspect of the threat posed by medical research comes from misguided or poorly regulated or ill intended bioengineering experiments to enhance the lethality of the world's most pathogenic viruses and bacteria. The purpose of this research is intended to anticipate the natural evolution of lethal pathogens so vaccines and other countermeasures can be developed to stop their potential release in the natural world. However, efforts to bioengineer improvements in the communicability and/or lethality of pathogens increase the potential risk they could escape biosafety laboratories and threaten public health. The US Government has the authority to approve medical and biological research involving any one of fifteen select agents. Unfortunately, the strength of any federally funded research depends on highly sophisticated biosafety controls that are often compromised by human factors. For example, errors in judgment, accidents, and even nefarious intentions can compromise the most secure biosafety laboratories in the world. Moreover, thousands of pathogens not subject to government oversight could be altered to create biological weapons and for this reason federal oversight of bioengineering research funded by the federal government is only a partial solution.

Above and beyond the federal government's list of dangerous pathogens, there are many naturally occurring novel pathogens that disperse through aerosol transmission without close contact. Viral pathogens like Covid-19 can be transmitted in aerosol form as far as twenty feet by individuals with especially forceful sneezes or coughs. Indeed, people with loud voices can discharge particles for much longer distances than the conventional wisdom of six feet. These individuals are called disease super-spreaders and they play an outsize role in accelerating the spread of disease.

Yet the greatest threats to humanity are less likely to come from bad actors in government biological research laboratories than from the natural evolution of existing highly communicable disease. Over time many pathogenic diseases have become more virulent, or what might be called a "gain of function" making them far more deadly than before a gain of function occurred. This process applies to literally billions of different species of viruses that exist on the planet including about 200 viruses that pose a threat to humanity—beyond those identified as select agents. When all species of infectious agents are counted, including viruses, bacteria, fungi, protozoa, and helminths, there are at least 1,415 known species that pose a threat of epidemic scale disease.

## 8.  Can future pandemics be prevented?

Future pandemics can be minimized but not prevented. The number of bacteria and viruses on this planet is so vast scientists have only speculated on the total number of species or the population of each species that exist in this world. Controlling our exposure to pathogens is a more realistic goal than one based on the wholesale elimination of every pathogen on the planet. Smallpox is the only highly lethal disease to have been eliminated from the world. That occurred in 1977 and the level of effort to remove smallpox from the inventory of pandemic disease took hundreds of thousands of public health workers more than seventy-five years of work including nearly ten years of intense coordinated international efforts to track down every case that remained in India, Africa, and the Middle East. This work was conducted by a rapid response team that used ring vaccination in tandem with quarantine to isolate the spread of smallpox village by village. Each village found to have smallpox was required to be vaccinated and stay put until active cases were no longer infectious. This approach was called ring vaccination since it created a ring of immunity that ensured the smallpox virus could not spread from one infected village to another. The work was undertaken under the sponsorship of the WHO and represents one of the greatest achievements of humanity. The chances such a public health campaign could be replicated for hundreds of other known pathogens is extremely unlikely.

While there are at least 1,415 species of infectious agents known to cause disease in humans, only 134 communicable diseases are well understood and considered public health concerns by the APHA. Lacking well-documented public health and medical treatment for over 1,281 infectious agents (i.e., 1,415 − 134 = 1,281) suggests the hope of eliminating these diseases rests on improved epidemiological studies of emerging and little studied pathogens. It would also require vast improvements to the public health, safety, and general welfare of the world's populations. Key strategies to minimize future pandemics will require (1) providing adequate shelter, drinkable water, and a wholesome diet for each person on the planet; (2) improving the surveillance of communicable disease throughout the world to ensure accurate information exists for pathogens that could trigger an epidemic; (3) tackling and reversing the destruction of ecosystems which serve as reservoirs for novel pathogens that pose a threat to humans when released to broader populations; (4) improving international coordination of emergency disease reporting; (5) expediting emergency response measures when an outbreak emerges; and (6) establishing enforceable sanctions for those nations that fail to adhere to WHO International Health Regulations.

The global effort to maintain the world's forests as habitat for a wide range of species facing extinction is not an environmental measure without benefit to human survival. Pandemic preparedness is made worse by the widespread loss of forest land since they play a critical role in maintaining a cooler climate and reducing the adverse impacts of fossil fuel emissions on the atmosphere. This in turn helps reduce human exposure to novel pathogens in many parts of the world. The release of carbon dioxide into the atmosphere creates the "greenhouse" effect thereby increasing temperatures on earth and in turn affecting the geographic range of highly communicable disease threatening human health. During the last century scientists have discovered more pathogenic diseases than were previously known to exist in the previous 2,000 years. Did these diseases exist in previous periods or does their existence represent our more sophisticated detection equipment capable of identifying pathogens by their genetic signatures. These are unanswered questions. However, we do know three to four new pathogenic viral and bacterial species are discovered annually and this by itself suggests our challenge in controlling communicable diseases will not be easy.

Another significant challenge to our ability to prevent future pandemics is the declining effectiveness of many antibiotics and antivirals formulated to treat highly communicable disease. Over time, bacteria and viruses mutate and antibiotics and antivirals lose their precious power to prevent disease including influenza, Covid-19, cholera, tuberculosis (TB), and food and waterborne disease such as Shigellosis and Salmonellosis. Our ability to stop the spread of tuberculosis will depend on the development of new antibiotics to counter the multi-drug resistant strains that have become common in many parts of the world. Significant progress was made in the early twentieth century to dramatically reduce cases and deaths from tuberculosis. However, by the late twentieth century the WHO found a significant uptick in TB cases. The WHO documented an estimated 1.4 to 2 million annual deaths from tuberculosis over the period 2000 to 2021 resulting in over 30 million deaths, making it the most lethal communicable disease in the world. Without treatment 60 percent of those infected with TB will die. Ironically, because TB is treated as an endemic disease, the public pays little attention to its threat. Many TB deaths are caused by multi-drug resistant strains, and this further complicates international efforts to eliminate it. Tuberculosis is so widespread the WHO estimates 25 percent of the world's population has been infected but most will not develop the disease, and some will clear the infection. With such an enormous reservoir of asymptomatic cases of TB in the world, the challenge of eliminating this disease is formidable.

Rather than stopping future epidemics, a more realistic goal will be to improve the immunological health of all people. By doing so we will be better prepared to handle the inevitable exposures we will face with an ever-expanding number of pathogens inhabiting a warming world. Furthermore, efforts to stop epidemic disease can't be made by each nation working in isolation from the public health measures undertaken in other nations. Coordinated international health measures must rely on evidence-based responses that have proven effective. The best available strategies must be applied wherever epidemic disease is found. Success in preventing communicable disease must start with a focus on those that have had the greatest impact on lives lost and the quality of life for those infected. This suggests, elimination of TB to be a priority international public health objective. The WHO concurs.

# How Epidemics and
# Pandemics Begin and Spread

## 9. How are epidemic diseases transmitted?

There are four principal ways epidemic disease gets transmitted into the human body: (1) inhalation, (2) ingestion, (3) injection, or (4) dermal contact. These are also called the portals of entry for disease and are distinct from the reservoirs where the pathogens reside. Airborne transmitted disease poses a particularly serious threat since it can be transmitted without close contact with an infected person or infectious agent. The small size of viral particles or bacteria facilitates their ability to stay suspended in air for long periods of time. For this reason, viral particles are of particular concern especially when an infected person shares the breathing zone with someone who has not yet been exposed to the disease. Exposure through inhalation may occur through droplets composed of viral particles aggregated with saliva discharged from the mouth of an infected person or they may be aggregated with dust particles suspended in the air. Droplet transmission is not ejected as far as the same particles released in a finer mist, or what is called an aerosol exposure.

Aerosol particles like those associated with the pathogen known as SARS-CoV-2 can be less than 5 microns in size. Particles of that size are not visible to the human eye. A micron is one millionth of a meter and a human hair can range from 17 to 90 microns. Imagine trying to see a viral particle that is at least 3 to 20 times smaller than the thickness of a human hair. Aerosol exposure is not merely a function of the size of the particle, but the time spent within its orbit. When an infected and exposed persons spend considerable time together—especially in an indoor environment with poor air circulation—the chances of inhaling an infectious dose increase enormously. These conditions are commonly found in many homes, restaurants, and bars where air circulation systems are either non-existent or provide less than optimal air changes to enable the rapid removal of contaminated air to the outside. The longer the exposure to a pathogenic aerosol the greater the number of infectious organisms capable of being inhaled. Diseases transmitted by aerosol exposure include tuberculosis, pneumonic plague, measles, pandemic flu, and Covid-19.

The second mode of transmission is through eating or drinking contaminated food or water. Cholera is transmitted by drinking water or eating uncooked food contaminated with the pathogen *Vibrio cholerae*. Similarly, Salmonella and typhoid are transmitted through eating contaminated and uncooked food. These diseases can infect thousands without adequate supplies of drinkable water or properly cleaned and cooked food. Food can also become contaminated by human or animal feces deposited near or upon agricultural crops prior to harvesting. In these cases, lack of sanitary controls over food processing have led to disease outbreaks. Boiling water is an important measure to eliminate exposure to waterborne diseases. For fruits and vegetables eaten in an uncooked state, thorough washing is essential to avoid foodborne pathogens. Epidemics caused by food and water can occur anywhere in the world but are especially a concern for third world nations lacking public water and sewer services.

Injection is the third mode of transmission and can occur in several ways. One means of exposure is through a bite of a mosquito. This form of transmission is associated with vector-borne disease. Several vector-borne diseases with the potential to create epidemic conditions include yellow fever, dengue, malaria, and Zika—all of which require transmission through the bite of a mosquito. The second way an injection can cause epidemic disease is through the use of contaminated needles. Doctors working in third world nations lacking an adequate supply of needles for vaccination or for drawing blood samples may reuse them without adequate sterilization. Indeed, because of the extremely high standards for needle sterilization, one time use of disposable needles is considered the best practice. Cases of Ebola have been transmitted from one person to another through the unfortunate practice of reusing improperly sterilized needles. Similarly, sharing common needles, heroin drug addicts have transmitted HIV/AIDS from one person to another without understanding the potential consequences. Exposure to diseases through injection may also occur by the bite of a rabies infected animal. Rabies is a communicable disease, but it rarely leads to widespread transmission to humans due to the existence of a rabies vaccine.

The fourth and last method of transmission is direct contact through dermal exposure such as kissing, sexual intercourse, touching pathogenic materials or hand to mouth transfer of pathogens. Handling contaminated food or washing one's hands in contaminated water can lead to exposure to such disease as cholera, typhoid, or Salmonella by hand to mouth transfer of these pathogens. Another means of exposure is directly through contact with infected animals or persons. Dermal exposure is the means for transmitting Monkeypox (recently renamed as Mpox), Ebola, and Marburg. An estimated 70 percent of all Mpox cases are attributable to contact with infected animals—and most recently by infected humans. In the case of Ebola and a related disease called Marburg, person-to-person transmission can occur through contact with infected blood, urine, vomit, or semen of someone recently infected. Airborne transmission has not been proven to occur with Ebola.

Ebola became a serious concern in America in 2014 when American nurses and physicians brought the disease back from Africa. While the disease did not spread in the United States, Ebola has a case fatality rate as high as 88 percent so even a modest level of infection triggers an epidemic level of public health response. Similarly, Marburg has a case fatality rate as high as 90 percent and poses similar concerns should any cases be identified in the United States. It is important to note an epidemic condition is not merely a function of how many are infected but the lethality of any given disease. Risk is based on the probability of exposure to any given disease times the severity of that potential exposure. In this context both Ebola and Marburg have severe life-threatening consequences raising cases of exposure to far higher levels of concern than diseases with much lower case fatality rates.

It is also important to distinguish between modes of transmission and the sources from which communicable diseases are transmitted. Communicable disease may originate from zoonotic sources such as rodents, primates, birds, pigs, etc. A second source of disease is from fomites, a term that refers to inanimate objects such as unsterilized medical equipment, a soiled napkin that has become contaminated by exposure to a pathogen or contact with soils laced with anthrax spores. Vectors are the third source of disease transmission, and this category includes fleas, rodents, mosquitoes, or wild geese. Finally, one of the most important concerns is exposure to aerosols. This can occur from exposure to suspended airborne pathogens or even from pathogens re-suspended off horizontal or vertical surfaces previously serving as pathogen reservoirs.

While there are four principal means of transmitting communicable disease, there are many diseases that, under certain conditions, may cause infection through more than one mode including plague (injection or inhalation); cholera (ingestion or dermal contact); Covid-19 (inhalation or dermal contact); anthrax (dermal contact or inhalation); human papillomavirus (sexual contact or through fomites). About 25 percent of the 1,415 species of infectious agents that are known to cause disease in humans have more than one mode of transmission. These examples underscore the importance of taking universal precautions when responding to novel pathogens where the modes of transmission are unknown.

## 10. How do epidemic diseases spread?

There are several factors that make it easier for disease to spread throughout a population. Highly congested living arrangements have often been a factor for spreading disease—especially those transmitted by inhalation. For example, in the nineteenth century Irish immigrants came to America on overcrowded vessels where dozens of people shared the same bunk space, the same eating utensils and common bathing and toilet facilities—all woefully inadequate to stop cholera and typhoid. Shared cutlery and food made it possible for diseases like cholera to infect many people simply because the food or water was contaminated with *Vibrio cholerae* the pathogen causing cholera. Similarly, diseases such as measles or tuberculosis are spread by spending a great deal of time in close contact with infected people.

Human behavior plays an enormous role in disease transmission. Individuals or communities with adequate nutrition, adequate shelter, sufficient income, and education are in a much better position to avoid contracting communicable disease. At a societal level, developed nations are more likely to have the resources and infrastructure to provide community public health services beyond basic human needs. Not all nations have sufficiently invested in hospital services, physician education, epidemic response programs, and basic public health education. Lacking these societal resources significantly impacts the overall health of any given underfunded nation state. Dozens of studies have linked the prevalence of infectious disease to a lack of nutrition, poor personal health, limited education, and poverty (McKeown, 1988). These factors increase susceptibility to communicable disease.

Inadequate nutrition is one of the most important factors that can compromise our immune system. In turn a compromised immune system makes us more susceptible to disease. Thomas McKeown was one of the first to recognize the role of improved nutrition as a key factor in the decline of infectious diseases in the twentieth century. Better nutrition improves immunity and that in turn minimizes the potential for infection. Eliminating extreme poverty is also an important strategy to reduce epidemics. Above and beyond improved nutrition, communicable disease can be prevented by expanding hygienic measures such as clean water, improved sewage disposal, improved food handling, and establishing minimum public health standards for habitable housing arrangements. These personal and public health practices have made an enormous difference in reducing the frequency and scale of epidemics in many developed nations. The absence of basic public health measures, extreme poverty, and limited education remain factors enabling epidemic disease in many nations of the world.

Another factor influencing the spread of airborne disease is technological in character. During the last 150 years, we have witnessed tighter seating arrangements in urban transit systems, theaters, airplanes, workrooms, stadiums, nursing homes, and many restaurants. Since space comes at a cost, the greater the capacity per square foot the greater the economic advantages of modern development. The unintended consequence of these business-driven decisions is to increase the potential exposure of healthy individuals to the pathogen laden exhalations of fellow workers, transit users, restaurant, or theater customers. While some of these exposure scenarios can be overcome by improved ventilation systems this is only one of several public health strategies needed to reduce the potential for epidemic-scale disease. Disease can also be transmitted through commonly shared objects such as doorknobs, handrails, subway transit poles, credit card readers, toilet seats and handles, library computer keyboards, shared cutlery, unwashed restaurant tables, coins and paper currency—sometimes called filthy lucre—and even library books on which a previous user recently sneezed.

Inadequate levels of air changes in restaurants, bars, or theaters have been associated with increased disease transmission of Covid-19. Whenever people spend extended periods of time in close contact with others, the chances for exposure to pathogens increase. One means of reducing airborne disease is not only to increase the air turnover rate inside buildings but to introduce ultraviolet light disinfection inside air vent systems. Ultraviolet light kills pathogens, and this can be accomplished out of sight of restaurant customers. Direct exposure to ultraviolet light is a safety and health hazard and therefore its use must be limited to air duct ventilation systems or similar non-habitable air spaces. Many hospitals rely on ultraviolet light disinfection to control airborne pathogens. Facilities that lack such infection control practices are more likely to harbor disease than those without such disinfection systems.

Modern standards of habitable space also directly influence the ease with which pathogens can be transmitted. The size of a bedroom influences exposure to aerosol pathogens. Larger rooms provide greater space between occupants and a larger volume of air to share amongst its users—both factors that attenuate exposure to airborne pathogens. Many nations have established minimum standards for habitable floor space with the express purpose of limiting the potential transmission of airborne disease. The American Public Health Association confirms bedrooms should not be less than 70 square feet and must not require access through another bedroom to reach a bathroom. One of the principles behind this standard is to reduce exposure to others who may be sick. For example, in nineteenth-century Boston, before the existence of public health standards for housing, as many as twenty-one families lived in one of the city's most crowded dwelling units. Extremely crowded living arrangements were frequently the source for the rapid spread of diseases like smallpox and cholera in nineteenth-century America.

## 11. How much of a pathogen is needed to create infection?

This is perhaps one of the most challenging questions to answer since one's susceptibility to any given disease will depend on the duration of exposure and the dose—as measured in colony forming units or virion particles per milliliter of air. The greater the dose, the longer the exposure duration and the closer the distance to the source of the pathogen the greater the chance of becoming infected. Dose, duration, and distance are also influenced by the health of the individual and his or her prior immunity to that disease. Moreover, two individuals could both have equal levels of exposure and dosage to the same pathogen yet react differently based on different levels of immunity. In one case, an individual may become infected and be diagnosed with clinical signs of disease while the other may be asymptomatic. This example demonstrates the challenge of establishing universal thresholds for what constitutes an infectious dose for any given pathogen.

From a practical perspective, universal precautions aim to eliminate exposure to any potential sources of disease. Counting the number of viral particles or bacteria that may exist on one's food or water or that might be floating in the air around us is simply not practical to avoid exposure. However, experimental investigations aimed at documenting pathogens in our food, water, or in the air are generally undertaken after an outbreak to confirm the need for public health interventions. Food processing facilities also rely on sampling to verify sanitation standards are effective and to mitigate instances where foodborne pathogens are identified. Bacteriological and viral sampling has been extensively used to develop infectious dose standards for a variety disease. These sampling initiatives are valuable for confirming the presence of pathogens in our food or water during an outbreak. Laboratory results alert the public of potential dangers of buying certain food products that may have been contaminated. Common examples include contamination by Salmonella, cholera, or typhoid. One study determined a Salmonella infectious dose could occur with fewer than 1,000 organisms—a quantity not visible to the naked eye.

Similar studies have also been conducted of exposure events during the Covid-19 pandemic to identify the range of virions needed to induce infection. For example, one recent study determined the threshold dose for a Covid-19 infection was an exposure to 300 to 2,000 virions for periods of 1 hour or longer. Not everyone exposed to these quantities of virions will become infected with Covid-19. People with greater immunity will require a larger exposure to the virus to contract the disease.

Cholera studies have determined ingestion of about 100 organisms can cause disease. Since virions are 1 to 3 microns in size—or twenty to 100 times smaller than the thickness of a human hair—it is not possible to see these pathogens on one's food or in the water. As a result, the only way to be sure one is not exposed to cholera is to diligently follow standard food preparation precautions. Be sure food is cleaned and cooked to temperatures that will kill the pathogens. It is unfortunate so many of us fail to appreciate our health until we fall ill. It is often after severe diarrhea, vomiting, fever, and being bed-ridden for days that we reflect back on what we might have eaten or failed to cook properly that led to our sickness. There are several other diseases including Norwalk virus and Salmonella that require very few organisms to produce illness. Both diseases can create illness through the ingestion of as few as ten organisms.

While many communicable diseases do not have established infectious dose standards, those that do are based on the principle that an infectious dose, called $ID_{50}$, means 50 percent of the people infected by the established dose will experience the infection. This approach allows public health professionals to quantify the dangers posed by any given disease to the population as a whole—not to any given individual.

## 12. What is a basic reproductive number?

The basic reproductive number (BRN) represents the rate of reproduction of a communicable disease pathogen over time. A disease with a high BRN with a short incubation period can spread quickly. The period between the time of exposure and the onset of infection is called the incubation period. The shorter the time between exposure and the onset of infection and the rapidity with which the pathogen can be transmitted can result in very high reproductive numbers. For example, measles is considered the world's most communicable disease. One of the reasons some disease is extremely contagious is because pathogens can be transmitted even before a person shows symptoms. A person infected with measles can infect other people four days before and after the appearance of clinical signs of disease. That means there are no outward signs of illness in the pre-symptomatic phase, so our natural instinct to protect ourselves are not activated. Normally we tend to take precautions when we know someone is sick. Measles is like the Trojan horse—it may appear innocuous because our friend looks well but he or she poses a significant threat to public health. Typically, measles has a BRN as high as 18—meaning each infected person can infect an additional eighteen persons. Each of those eighteen persons, in turn can transmit the disease to eighteen more people and with this ongoing rate of transmission measles can quickly become an epidemic.

However, it is important to understand diseases with long incubation periods such as tuberculosis can also have a relatively high BRN of 8. The explanation is that the BRN is not measuring the speed of infection but simply the rate of reproduction of the pathogen amongst a susceptible population. TB infected persons can infect as many as eight other people even though the disease may take up to ten weeks after exposure before symptoms appear. For this reason, it is possible to have fast- and slow-moving epidemics because the rate of transmission is not an element of the BRN. The BRN simply measures how many secondary cases are created from an infected person. A long incubation period, such as that for TB or HIV/AIDS, tends to gather less public attention because humans are hard wired to respond to immediate threats—not slow-moving ones.

A BRN reflects both the biological aspects of the pathogen and the environmental, geographic, and social and behavioral characteristics of the impacted population (see question 10). As used by epidemiologists the BRN reflects the contagiousness of a disease as it impacts a susceptible population with no prior immunity to that disease. For many diseases, where prior immunity exists in some segments of the population, the term used is the "effective reproductive number" since prior exposure or immunity through vaccination alters the contagiousness of the disease (see question 19). BRNs are always calculated after epidemics have ended—or in some cases after the first wave of an epidemic. Yet the ever-frenzied media world is fed by overanxious epidemiologists and medical scientists rushing to shed light on the threat posed by a pandemic. In these instances, epidemiologists will generate BRN numbers for (1) individual outbreaks within a pandemic, (2) short segments of time within an epidemic, (3) emergent variant phases of an epidemic, or (4) even country level BRNs simply to track unique density, cultural, behavioral, or ethnological perspectives on disease transmission. The validity and utility of these micro-scale investigations for pandemic response planning is subject to some debate.

Studies that indicate the contagiousness of a disease, say a BRN of 18 for measles, cannot be applied to other outbreaks of measles without understanding the range of environmental social and biological factors that have changed since the previous epidemic. It is critical to understand a BRN is highly dependent on population densities, climate, geography, transportation systems, and public wellness of the population affected. A BRN for measles calculated for a third world nation without basic access to public health services, adequate nutrition, and shelter—living in highly overcrowded living arrangements— will likely be far higher than the same measles outbreak in a rural area of the Midwestern United States. In effect, the BRN is not an inherent biological feature of the pathogen but represents an interplay of its biological features—including its ease of transmission—with the environment and behavior of the exposed population.

While the use of BRN has become more common in recent epidemics—such as that of Covid-19—there is often a great deal of misunderstanding concerning its meaning when applied to an epidemic or a specific wave within an epidemic. Rarely, do media reports qualify the use of the BRN within the context of the public health, economic, social, and housing conditions of any given nation for which a number is assigned. By definition, every epidemic will have a BRN of more than 1. An important purpose in estimating the number of secondary cases ensuing from each infected case is to increase public awareness of how easy it is to get infected and to bring the resources to bear to counter its continued spread.

# 13. What is an incubation period and how can it affect the spread of an epidemic disease?

An incubation period is the time interval between the first contact with the disease and the onset of symptoms associated with the infection. For vector-borne diseases, the incubation period is measured from the time the organism enters the vector—for example, a mosquito—and the time when the vector can transmit the infection. A vector incubation period is called an extrinsic incubation period because the pathogen operates for part of its life cycle outside the human body.

Diseases that have a very short incubation period—the plague, measles, cholera—are diseases that pose the greatest threat of triggering an epidemic. Plague has an incubation period from one to seven days; measles has an average incubation period of fourteen days and cholera usually has an incubation period of two to three days. Susceptible persons who come into contact with people infected with one of these diseases—or the vectors for the disease in the case of plague—can become infected. Because of the short incubation periods for these diseases, an outbreak can quickly become an epidemic. The rapidity by which a pathogen is transmitted across networks of friends, family, and co-workers can expand the disease from patient zero to hundreds of others. Even more causal contacts that might happen at theaters, bars, gyms, restaurants can also serve as opportunities for disease transmission—especially for pathogens with a low infectious dose.

At the other extreme, tuberculosis and HIV/AIDS have very long incubation period. The onset of disease can be as long as ten weeks in the case of tuberculosis and as long as ten to fifteen years for AIDS. The result of these extended incubation periods before the onset of disease is that these epidemics tend to get less immediate attention, resources, and public health interventions. In many respects, humans are hard wired to respond to immediate threats to life and limb and are less concerned with disease with a long incubation period. Yet tuberculosis represents the most lethal epidemic of the twenty-first century with over 30 million deaths worldwide. Similarly, the World Health Organization (WHO) estimates 40.1 million died from AIDS since the epidemic began in the 1970s. The relatively limited public attention given to these two unsung and undeclared pandemics reflects their mind numbingly long period for the manifestation of symptoms.

For some communicable disease, the incubation period may also be a period where the infected person can transmit the disease to others—unbeknownst to the innocent victim. This is an especially significant factor in accelerating the spread of disease since there are no outward signs a person is infected. In turn, this means one's natural tendency to avoid sick people is not activated. Lacking any concern for personal exposure simplifies the germ's goal of getting more people infected. From this perspective, measles is one of the most dangerous diseases on the planet. Those exposed to measles but not yet showing clinical signs of disease play a significant role in its rapid transmission.

## 14. What is a disease's infectious period and how can it influence an epidemic?

A disease infectious period occurs when a pathogen is capable of being transmitted to others. The infectious period often begins at the first symptoms of infection and lasts for a period usually prior to the elimination of symptoms. However, some diseases like measles, mumps, rubella, pertussis, influenza, AIDS, and several others can be infectious prior to the onset of symptoms. Diseases that have a significant percentage of the infectious period overlapping with the incubation period pose significant challenge for public health officials. In these instances, children could be attending school and appear perfectly healthy without any symptoms of disease and be contagious. Imposing stay at home orders becomes more complicated in these instances because school nurses or physicians will have no way of telling whether any given child is infected. For highly communicable disease, some school superintendents may take precautionary measures to close an entire school or a specific classroom out of the abundance of caution.

Perhaps the most valuable outcome of improved testing may be the opportunity to identify cases of infection prior to onset of symptoms. Obviously, such an approach can be controversial as well as expensive. PCR testing procedures can be used to identify the presence of pathogens before the onset of symptoms. However, these tests are expensive and require the cooperation of the parents of the children. This is an emerging area of public and occupational health practice that has not developed standardized protocols. This strategy is unlikely to see the light of day due to the overly intrusive testing it would require of so-called healthy people.

Yet, early testing or pre-emptive stay at home orders can make the difference between an outbreak that is quickly stopped and one spiraling out of control.

Improved testing, contact tracing, and stay at home orders play a critical role in the control of communicable disease. These measures depend upon much more inclusive and plain English strategies for explaining the importance of community and family support for early interventions. Early diagnosis is extremely important in the case of HIV/AIDS. This disease complex can take years for symptoms to appear even though persons infected can transmit the pathogen far earlier. Failure to understand the infectious period for any given disease can result in reactive responses that occur far too late to stop an outbreak. The result is the outbreak spirals into a full-scale epidemic—as has occurred with HIV/AIDS. Not knowing the degree to which the infectious period overlaps with the incubation period of the disease makes it difficult to initiate timely public health countermeasures such as vaccination, sanitation, universal health precautions, and restrictions on human behavior. Waiting for symptoms to appear in children in a school age population, when at least one measles case has been identified, can mean a loss of up to a week's time in responding to an outbreak. For these reasons, asymptomatic disease transmission represents the greatest challenge to stopping epidemics.

One of the least understood but significant infectious period is that in the post-symptomatic phase of disease. There are many examples of people who have contracted diseases like typhoid or even Covid-19 and remain infectious even after their symptoms have disappeared. The most famous example is that of Typhoid Mary, an Irish cook who lived in New York City in the early nineteenth century. She contracted typhoid and recovered from her illness. However, she continued to work as a cook and infected dozens of people who ate her food or came into contact with her. She was the prototype super-spreader of typhoid. She remained a healthy woman with no visible symptoms and yet she continued to carry the typhoid pathogen within her (see question 18). Post-symptomatic cases of infection are not as unusual as some may think. Some disease remains latent within us and only appear when our immunity is compromised.

## 15. Why do diseases mutate over time, and how does this affect the spread of epidemics?

Diseases can mutate in several ways including through random changes in the genetic makeup of the organism—whether virus or bacterium. For example, e-coli can double in quantity in 20 minutes resulting in 4.7 sextillions organisms in 24 hours or equivalent to $2^{22}$ cell divisions. With this rate of cell divisions, it does not take long for bacteria to mutate. It only takes billions of cell divisions, or about $2^{10}$ cell divisions for any given pathogen to improperly replicate its DNA or RNA sequences. The result can either make the pathogen more or less able to infect its host—or the mutation may have no impact at all.

Mutations compromise the integrity of vaccines. Whenever a pathogen mutates the original vaccine may no longer be effective. For example, there are two strains of cholera, referred to as serogroups 01 and 0139. Infection from cholera serogroup 01 does not provide immunity to serogroup 0139. This means herd immunity is lost when a new cholera strain emerges or when a previous vaccine is no longer effective.

Mutations of the bacterium *Mycobacterium tuberculosis* created multi-drug resistant strains and these strains now represent a major threat to human health. According to the WHO, without treatment 50 percent of those infected die. However, when treatment is available as many as 85 percent of those infected can be cured. The number of multi-drug resistant strains has increased in recent years with over 450,000 cases in 2022. Because of this problem the WHO has indicated that multi-drug and extremely multi-drug resistant TB only achieved a 60 percent treatment success rate in 2019. If multi-drug resistant TB continues to evade available antibiotic options, WHO efforts to eliminate this disease by 2025 are unlikely.

One of the most significant public health risks is posed by the ease with which genetic material can be transferred between bacterial species. In this case the transfer of plasmids, a component of bacteria's cellular structure, can replicate and transfer to other bacteria. This process enables a relatively quick transfer of antibiotic-resistant features across different bacteria. The transfer of plasmids can occur where there is a "broth of bacteria" such as in wastewater treatment plants, contaminated rivers and lakes, and similar environments. The discharge of antibiotics down the toilet or sink ends up in wastewater treatment plants. Once discharged into rivers, these wastewaters contain a potpourri of pathogens and discarded drugs. The presence of discarded antibiotics can selectively enhance the growth of bacteria resistant to a wide range of antibiotics tossed down the drain. Rather than dispose of antibiotics in this fashion, there are many cities and pharmacies that have developed collection programs to avoid these unfortunate witches brew of highly drug-resistant bacteria in the nation's rivers and waters.

When viral or bacterial pathogens are no longer prevented by vaccines or antibiotics, germs will have a field day at our expense. Human adaptation to disease is not something that happens in 24 hours or twenty-four years.

It takes multiple-multiple generations and tens of thousands of years to adapt to ever mutating pathogens. By that time, the original bacteria or virus would have undergone far-far more than trillions of mutations. We cannot keep up with the threats posed by pathogens through genetic or natural mutations of our human DNA. Clearly our inability to adapt genetically at the speeds which viruses and bacteria mutate means we must (1) focus on protecting the integrity of existing antibiotics and vaccines, (2) develop new antibiotics and vaccines, and (3) develop more effective public health strategies to address the root causes of epidemic disease.

## 16. What factors increase susceptibility to epidemic disease?

Susceptibility to disease can be associated with activities falling within our own span of control and those influenced by broader activities carried out at the community, national, and international levels.

Six things increase our susceptibility to epidemic disease and fall within our span of control. Whenever, an approved vaccine exists for an epidemic disease, our failure to get vaccinated increases our susceptibility to infection. The efficacy of vaccines varies enormously depending on the disease and the vaccine. The Food and Drug Administration (FDA) is charged with approving vaccines based on rigorous studies to ensure their efficacy. The FDA also is tasked with determining the types and frequency of their adverse effects. In those instances where adverse effects are identified, the vaccines will come with notifications and restrictions on their use to individuals with allergies or other anticipated adverse reactions.

A second significant susceptibility factor to epidemic-scale disease is our failure to keep healthy. This is a major cause of disease for the elderly or individuals not getting a proper diet or exercise. For example, those with preexisting health conditions such as obesity, diabetes, chronic obstructive pulmonary disease, smoking, alcoholism, and similar ailments compromise immunity. As such they are much more likely to become infected than those in peak fitness. In many countries of the world, poor nutrition or a lack of food are contributing factors influencing susceptibility to epidemic capable disease. Higher measles case fatality rates are found in nations or refugee camps where lack of food, water, and shelter compromise immune systems.

A third factor is living with severe stress environments, typical of the hustle and bustle of modern life, also affect our immune system. Given these predisposing factors, spending considerable amounts of time in crowded environments also increases our exposure and therefore our susceptibility to aerosol pathogens. These environments also increase the chances of exposure to unknown pathogens for which prior immunity is not likely. A fourth factor increasing our susceptibility to epidemic disease is simply by failing to follow public health precautions. It is not uncommon for the younger generation, to act as immortals and dismiss public health recommendations as not applicable. Public health education must be an integral part of civics education and be offered at all levels of the educational system. This remains a work in progress.

At a community level, there are several factors that make communities or nations more susceptible to epidemic disease. High poverty levels, overcrowded housing, poor ventilation systems in public and private buildings, and tightly packed transit systems increase the chances individuals will be exposed to an epidemic-scale disease. Similarly, limited public investment in monitoring, reporting, and responding to outbreaks makes an entire community or nation more susceptible to an epidemic. If it isn't measured, it is not managed, and this principle is a foundation stone for all successful epidemic response measures.

Finally, there is insufficient skilled staff at hospitals, public health agencies, and even within all levels of the public education system. Right understanding leads to right action and this is a basic principle underlying the need for public health education. Governmental investments in medical and public health education directly influence our overall susceptibility to disease. Lacking public education increases the likelihood errors in judgment will be made. Finally, lack of adequate and affordable housing is a public good. It not only protects the health of the homeless and those living from paycheck to paycheck—it supports the health of the entire population. Yet those of us lucky enough to have housing are not immune from disease. Each of us can be exposed to disease simply by our collective failure to meet the housing needs of our most vulnerable populations. Those without housing and forced to live in crowded shelters for the homeless are more vulnerable to epidemic scale disease. These housing conditions, in turn, make it possible for disease to infect everyone within the community—even the rich and those with suitable shelter. Disease connects all of us. How many of us know of people living on the street or in their car because they simply don't have the financial resources to rent or buy a home? Their health affects our health and their susceptibility to disease may come full circle. In an interconnected world, the most susceptible may be the entry point for infecting an entire community.

# 17. What is a super-spreader and what role do they play in epidemics?

A super spreading event (SSE) is defined as a transmission event involving an unusually large number of cases, initiated by an individual termed a super-spreader. To be called a super-spreader one must be capable of transmitting greater quantities of pathogens than the norm. Super-spreader may also have exceptional social skills. Such skills may include spending time in crowded buildings in close quarters with other people on a routine basis. Diseases transmitted by aerosols are of particular concern as they are transmitted longer distances and stay airborne for longer times than disease where transmission is through droplets. Three basic factors determine who are most likely to be super-spreader amongst the population of infected persons; those with loud voices including singers capable of projecting their voices over long distances; individuals with social networking skills that bring them into contact with many other people; and those who participate in close contact events such as activities at schools, funerals, weddings, conferences, gymnasiums, and similar events. While many of us may think we meet these super-spreader criteria because of our social skills, not everyone has the ability to easily spew out viral or bacterial particles while speaking in a conversational tone of voice.

The general rule of thumb developed by some scientists is super-spreaders are responsible for 80 percent of disease transmission yet represent 20 percent or less of the population of infected individuals. SSEs can also be influenced by the stage of infection. The quantity of virions that may be expelled from the mouth of a super-spreader not only is influenced by whether he or she is breathing, speaking, or singing—each of which has different levels of viral transmission—it is also influenced by his or her viral or bacterial load. The optimum time for the transmission of some diseases may occur several days before symptoms appear—as in the case of measles—and for other diseases the most infectious period is just when symptoms appear. For diseases such as measles, where asymptomatic transmission is a concern, super-spreaders pose a clear and present danger to public health. How would one know an individual is a super-spreader if they show no signs of disease? This suggests, absent any symptoms of disease with those we spend time, the only smart choice might be staying out of crowded places, avoiding close contact with others, and wearing a face mask. Of course, this would be a drastic solution for many people living in the modern world. Life is full of risks and the best course of action is to be an informed citizen and recognize the public health dangers that exist in our community.

Super-spreaders are often the most sociable and highly networked individuals at any given party or event. Their natural ability to communicate with all sorts of people makes it possible for such individuals to play an outsized role in disease transmission. An example of one super-spreader event occurred in December 2020. At that time, Santa Claus visited a home care facility in Belgium and infected 100 residents and forty staff members resulting in twenty-six deaths from Covid-19. This example underscores how one person, who was the center of attention for hundreds of people in the audience, became a super-spreader of disease. One factor contributing to super-spreader events includes the susceptibility of the people infected—especially elderly and immune compromised individuals. Elderly persons living in nursing homes and assisted living facilities experienced very high rates of Covid-19 infection. This was partly due to their weaker immune system. Another factor was close contact with nursing aides and other support staff who failed to use face masks or social distancing practices. In this instance, the super-spreader events were strongly influenced by close contact and crowded congregant facilities. Nursing staff did not need any exceptional networking skills or any special biological or voice projection abilities to infect thousands of immunocompromised elderly. In this context, super-spreader events are influenced by both the super-spreader's ability to eject large doses of pathogens further than others as well as by the number of exposed immunocompromised persons. It takes two to tango when anticipating the worst-case scenario for the rapid transmission of disease. A super-spreader might be called a "professional cougher or sneezer" or an individual with exceptional voice projection skills. Yet these skills need not be performing at the highest level of projection when he or she stands before a highly susceptible group of immunocompromised souls.

## 18. What does it mean to be asymptomatic, and can an asymptomatic person spread disease?

An asymptomatic person does not exhibit or produce symptoms of disease. For diseases like mumps, German measles, chickenpox, measles, and the poliovirus, exposed individuals can infect others even without visible signs of illness. Pathogens capable of being transmitted during the incubation phase are of great public health concern. Neither the infected person nor those in close contact during the asymptomatic phase will be aware of the public health risk this situation poses.

There are two ways asymptomatic individuals pose a risk to public health. The first case is what is called the pre-symptomatic phase before any symptoms of disease appear. In these instances, the individual may shed pathogens for a brief period before the full symptoms of disease appear. Some studies have suggested this pre-symptomatic phase may have accounted for as much as 30 percent of all the Covid-19 infections during the first two years of the pandemic. This was never known at the outset of the pandemic—an unfortunate and costly lesson learned.

The second way an infected person without symptoms poses a public health risk is after recovery from their illness. Some people recover but continue to shed pathogens thereby infecting other people. This is called the post symptomatic phase and was made famous by Typhoid Mary, whose real name was Mary Mallon. She was infected with typhoid during her years as a New York City cook. She never recovered from typhoid and yet she never exhibited any symptoms of disease throughout her life. Cases like that of Typhoid Mary underscore the importance of detecting and treating those who appear perfectly healthy based on symptoms but continue to be contagious. In Typhoid Mary's case she was placed in quarantine for the rest of her life—a draconian strategy that was chosen after she failed to follow public health edicts to stop working as a cook. In her defense, she was a poor Irish woman who had no other occupational skills or interests and needed to work to survive. In her role as cook she continued to infect many people who ate the food she prepared—including some who died.

Mary Mallon's case underscores the importance of broad testing to identify contagious individuals who continue to pose a threat to public health. Identifying pre-symptomatic or post-symptomatic cases is expensive but a necessary testing strategy to understand the public health burdens created by asymptomatic carriers of disease. Yet there must be limits to over-intrusive public health measurements. Treatments and testing must be consistent with modern public health commitments to minimize harm to the person undergoing treatment or testing. The Typhoid Mary case is an extreme case of government overreach. Yet Typhoid Mary was also an extreme example of a person unwilling or unable to adjust her life and cooking profession to avoid infecting others. When a person becomes a lethal weapon, by dint of their highly infectious nature, there are societal consequences for such behavior.

The scale of asymptomatic infection within the world's population is not known. Yet this is a significant factor in the transmission of disease between apparently healthy individuals and sectors of the community that have compromised immune systems. An asymptomatic person can transmit pathogens at doses that may not be infectious to a healthy person but may be sufficient to trigger disease in those with compromised health. This represents an ongoing threat to the most vulnerable populations in the world. Those most at risk are the elderly, those confined in prisons, or with HIV/AIDS and tuberculosis. Compromised immune systems whether caused by age, infirmity, or medical interventions are enablers for super-spreader killing fields.

## 19. Is there a natural progression for an epidemic disease? Will an epidemic or pandemic eventually die out on its own?

No, there is not one natural progression for an epidemic disease. Many diseases have the potential to become epidemics but may be quickly controlled through available vaccines or through rapid interventions. Prompt public health interventions can limit the spread within the community. Yet without intervention a communicable disease has the potential to become an epidemic. In practical terms, this means an infected person can pass the disease onto at least two additional persons each of whom can pass it on to at least two more persons. At any point in this process, it is possible to intervene. Depending upon the communicability of the disease there are various public health measures that should be considered.

In an ideal world, if a vaccine exists for an epidemic-scale disease, then it should be introduced as soon as sufficient supplies are available to protect the susceptible population. Unfortunately, there are many communicable diseases for which vaccines do not exist. This is especially the case for novel pathogens that have never been seen before—for example Covid-19. Where vaccines and medical treatments are either non-existent or in short supply, the emphasis shifts to what is called non-pharmaceutical solutions. This starts by isolating infected individuals, so the novel pathogen is contained. Secondly, those who may have been exposed to an infected person should be quarantined. The quarantine period is normally the maximum length of the incubation period for the disease. However, the quarantine may be shortened if an individual shows one or more symptoms. In these instances, the infected person is now subject to isolation procedures mentioned above.

In a world where pathogens travel unchecked without human effort to intervene, epidemic disease can spread rapidly. However, human intervention, of one kind or another almost always occurs. Interventions are triggered by medical evidence of disease but sometimes through word of mouth. The media also plays a role in the evolution of an epidemic. Deadly threats awaken our sense of mortality, and the media is expert in showcasing the three Ds—death, disease, and disaster. Invoking these gods of fear inevitably triggers a demand for a rapid public health response. This in turn influences the natural progression of disease—sometimes in the wrong direction. When the public learns they are living at the epicenter of an epidemic the natural response is often to flee. The unintended consequence of this behavior disperses lethal pathogens far and wide. In this context, fear, and the desire to flee the epicenter of the epidemic facilitate the natural progression of disease.

One public health intervention that has had a profound impact on altering the natural progression of disease is contact tracing. The purpose of contact tracing is to identify persons who might have been exposed to infected individuals. Rather than a disease progressing to infect everyone in the population, a well-organized contact tracing program can quickly identify and quarantine potential carriers of disease. When done properly, it can slow or stop the natural progression of disease.

In recent years, with advances in genomic testing for pathogens, it is now possible to also determine who may have been exposed to a disease even before he or she has visible symptoms. Early testing is critical for individuals with communicable disease, like Covid-19 and measles. Individuals infected with these two diseases can infect others even before exhibiting symptoms. The existence of asymptomatic carriers of disease makes it far more challenging to stop these epidemics. In these cases, genetic or antibody testing of apparently healthy individuals serves as a complementary measure to refine the application of contact tracing. When people who appear healthy are transmitting disease, visual clues to determine the need for treatment or quarantine are useless. Fortunately, genetic testing has made it possible to identify people who appear healthy but are carriers. Asymptomatic carriers play an outsized role in disease transmission. This is a major innovation in public health practice that has emerged in the last twenty years. It augurs well for changing the natural progression of disease.

If these public health interventions are unable to stop the natural progression of disease, then there is a greater likelihood the outbreak will lead to an epidemic. Absent vaccines or other medical prophylaxis, the disease can infect the entire susceptible population. In these instances, everyone will either get sick and recover or die. Those who recover will have immunity. The level of immunity varies by disease. In the case of highly mutable variants of Covid-19, immunity may only last several months or more. In the case of measles, immunity lasts a lifetime. By achieving herd immunity, a disease dies out for lack of susceptible persons to infect. The number of persons who must be infected and recover varies by the BRN for that disease (see question 12). In essence the more easily the disease can be transmitted the greater the percentage of the population that must become immune before the epidemic stops. Immunity may be achieved by prior infection, or it may be acquired through vaccination when available. For novel pathogens like Covid-19, the disease's natural progression may have been more likely if there had not been the spectacular creation of the first ever vaccine developed and deployed in the heat of the pandemic.

There is a saying, diseases don't die they just become endemic. While this is technically not true—smallpox was eradicated from the world in 1977—all other known communicable diseases remain active in one or more reservoirs in the world. There are two diseases on a high priority list for elimination—tuberculosis and measles—both of which the WHO believes could be removed from the list of pandemic diseases if the nations of the world commit the resources and time to do so.

# Combatting Epidemics and Pandemics

## 20. In the United States, who is in charge of organizing a response to an epidemic?

The organizations responsible for a response to an epidemic depends on the origin of the disease, its threat to public health or national security and the relevant laws and regulations governing the response. Typically, outbreaks of "home grown" diseases will be managed by state public health agencies in coordination with county or municipal health departments affected by the outbreak (see question 4). In contrast, epidemics that are imported from other nations carried into America by infected passengers or contaminated goods will initially be managed by the Centers for Disease Control and Prevention (CDC) and the US Department of Health and Human Services. Because of the divided public responsibilities for epidemic response in America, the CDC is only authorized to respond to interstate transmission of disease and those entering the nation through its borders. The laws governing the interstate transmission of disease allows the CDC to regulate interstate transportation to minimize, if not stop, the spread of disease. However, the CDC is not authorized to intervene in state public health matters. In this context, the CDC, a major operating arm of the Department of Health and Human Services, is only able to influence state-level epidemic response measures through the power of the federal purse strings. The CDC's influence is also a function of the power of its world class epidemic intelligence service. The expression that is apropos in this context has long been "When the CDC talks, everyone listens." The CDC has long been an international center of public health excellence, and this has enabled it to provide leading edge advice to state-level epidemic response teams. This, of course, broke down during the Covid-19 pandemic and revealed the degree to which the agency was consumed with getting all the facts before making any decisions—a bias associated with its more academic approach to emergencies. The culture of the CDC emphasized certainty before action, which resulted in paralysis (Lessons from the Covid War, The Covid Crisis Group, 2023). The CDC's ability to influence public policy was further marginalized when the Trump administration abdicated responsibility for pandemic planning. While this was unfortunate, it was not the first example of the agency's flat-footed response to an epidemic. One of the lessons from Covid-19 is that no one can be prepared for a novel pathogen for which no prior scientific or medical knowledge existed.

Epidemics can also be a threat to national security. In this context, the anthrax crisis was an example of a disease that had a relatively limited impact on public health but significant adverse impact on the security of federal, state, and local governments. Many government agencies in Washington, DC, were closed for extended periods of time due to anthrax laced letters sent to senators and inadvertently distributed to dozens of other government facilities in the area. The military took an active interest in the anthrax crisis since there was some evidence the perpetrators could have been connected to the 9/11 terrorists who hijacked three domestic airline flights two of which crashed into the World Trade Center and the Pentagon in Washington, DC. While this link has never been proven—largely because the 9/11 perpetrators are now dead—there was enough evidence to trigger military investigations. One of the outcomes of the anthrax crisis has been a far greater military commitment to tracking bioterrorism threats across the world—particularly those with a connection to national security.

When an outbreak of disease occurs in America, there may be multiple responsible organizations depending on the threat posed, the location of the outbreak and the legal authority to intervene. In many cases—especially when an outbreak involves a highly lethal select agent—there may be multiple federal and state public health, military, and law enforcement agencies working in tandem. In this context, an effective epidemic response should rely on the playbooks established by the National Incident Management System under the authority of the Department of Homeland Security. Specifically, a Unified Incident Command Structure is best suited for a coordinated multi-agency epidemic response. This approach was effectively used during the anthrax response in 2001/2002. However, it was not used in the Covid-19 response— which explains, in part, the dysfunctional and uncoordinated response measures adopted across the nation. There was no single standardized approach to the Covid-19 response adopted across the fifty states or overseas territories. The ever-changing rules issued by state governments made it difficult for the public to have confidence in public health orders or recommendations. Moreover, the ongoing policy changes in one state's Covid-19 playbook were almost always different than those of every other state. For example, more than 400 different face mask rules were issued by the fifty states and territories over the first two years of the pandemic. The rapidity of policy changes in when, where, and why to wear a mask led to ineffectual communication strategies. The ongoing face mask policy changes made it clear those in charge had lost touch with the basic communication principle of keeping the message short and simple. Given these "wild-west" Covid-19 policies found across the United States, will a unified command structure be possible?

A Unified Incident Command Structure is not easy to activate but represents the most effective means of coordinating epidemics and pandemics that cross state and regulatory boundaries. Few federal and state public agencies are well educated in this coordinated intergovernmental command structure. The expert in the use of Unified Incident Command is the US Forest Service. They are the world's leaders in the use of coordinated multi-agency responses conducted to control mega fires crossing state lines. Like forest fires that consume all the dry wood in its path, pandemics burn through the susceptible population until everyone is infected or dies. In this context, the long-term value of a unified command system will depend upon extensive training and education of public health professionals at all levels of government. It will also require new federal legislation that places a premium on intergovernmental cooperation.

## 21. What institutions are responsible for global responses to pandemics?

There are a wide range of organizations responsible for global response to pandemics. Indeed, there are a hierarchy of responsibilities that are brought to bear in the case of pandemics. For example, pandemics require advanced planning and investments to prepare for the eventuality of fast spreading disease. Once a pandemic condition has been declared, a range of organizations are responsible for monitoring, reporting, responding, and caring for those exposed and infected.

The primary institution responsible for a global pandemic response is the World Health Organization (WHO). The WHO is composed of 196 member nations each of which has voluntarily adopted the WHO's International Health Regulations. The WHO monitors communicable disease outbreaks with the aid of member nations and related private sector partners. Because of many shortcomings in the world-wide response to Covid-19, over 110 nations, including the European Union, have called for a new international treaty on pandemic prevention and preparedness under the authority of the WHO. While a new treaty will not change the overall role of the WHO, it is likely to establish new standards for member nations reflecting the lessons learned from Covid-19.

Many nations, including China, the European Union, and the United States have independently undertaken their own international disease monitoring and public health interventions. For example, the US CDC provides technical assistance, when requested, for nations experiencing an outbreak. A case in point is the CDC's international pandemic response program known as the Global Health Security Agenda. This initiative addresses the public health needs for over sixty member nations. The CDC has also invested in public health readiness for nineteen nations seeking help with developing emergency preparedness centers. These centers are designed to detect and respond to emerging infectious disease.

Similarly, the United States Agency for International Development, known by the acronym USAID, has provided more than a billion dollars in support for Global Health Security—a program complementing the work of the CDC. The USAID also partners with the US Department of State, US Department of Health and Human Services, and other federal departments and agencies to implement the Global Health Security Agenda.

The CDC also is responsible for tracking zoonotic disease throughout the world. This work is conducted by the CDC's National Center for Emerging and Zoonotic Infectious Diseases. The Center is responsible, among other duties, for protecting people from global threats such as (1) foodborne and waterborne illnesses; (2) infections spread in hospitals; (3) infections resistant to antibiotics; (4) deadly diseases like Ebola and anthrax; (5) illnesses that affect immigrants, migrants, refugees, and travelers; (6) disease caused by contact with animals; and (7) disease carried by mosquitoes, ticks, and fleas.

Perhaps the most important American effort to enhance pandemic response capabilities is that created by the Biden administration. In September 2021, President Biden called for a sweeping overhaul of the nation's pandemic response efforts. In October 2022, the Biden administration released its *National Biodefense Strategy and Implementation Plan*. That plan placed responsibility for emergency preparedness and pandemic response under an organization known as Administration for Strategic Preparedness and Response (ASPR). ASPR is a branch of the US Department of Health and Human Services but functions in cooperation with multiple coordinating federal agencies. While no additional funding has been allocated for this effort, the most significant aspect of this initiative is its removal of the CDC as the primary actor in the nation's pandemic response measures. The objective of the ASPR reflects its origin. Its mission is a response to the nation's failure to properly plan and control the Covid-19 pandemic.

The military sectors of the federal government also play important roles in pandemic surveillance and response measures. For example, the Defense Threat Reduction Agency and the Armed Forces Health Surveillance Center both have significant expertise in tracking, disease diagnostics, and treatment regimens for biological threats to the United States. Ever since the anthrax attacks of 2001, the military has placed great emphasis on bio-warfare threats and weapons of mass destruction. Their expertise is part of America's expanding ability to respond to international outbreaks of disease.

Like the United States, Canada's Public Health plays an important role in the pandemic early warning system. Its Global Public Health Intelligence Network monitors internet activity to provide advance intelligence of emerging disease. This Canadian initiative is an integral part of the WHO's Global Outbreak Alert and Response Network.

In addition, there are at least five private sector initiatives essential to global pandemic response. For example, the Bill & Melinda Gates Foundation provides funding for the control of four tropical diseases: Chagas, leprosy, sleeping sickness, and Leishmaniosis. It has also funded efforts to eliminate polio under the WHO's Global Polio Eradication Initiative (GPEI) and invested $2 billion in the fight against Covid-19. Similarly, the Rockefeller Foundation's Pandemic Prevention Initiative focuses on research and funding for vaccination strategies to control the Covid-19 pandemic. The foundation also commits resources for a wide range of public health initiatives throughout the world. A third non-profit organization, the Skoll Global Threat Fund, underwritten by billionaire Jeffrey Skoll, addresses strategies to predict and prevent pandemics and provides funding to achieve these objectives. A fourth, Global Solutions for Infectious Diseases, is a non-profit organization located in California with expertise in vaccine development. It was founded in 2004 and focuses on disease surveillance and the development of vaccines for infectious disease. Finally, the Global Alliance for Vaccine and Immunization, GAVI, is a non-profit organization with a mission to provide vaccines for communicable disease to the world's susceptible population. It is funded by the Bill & Melinda Gates Foundation and supported by the WHO and the World Bank to name a few of the major benefactors for this initiative. GAVI's role in fighting communicable disease through vaccines is a critical element in pandemic response planning. It directly funds nations across the planet in need of vaccine resources during pandemics.

The World Bank also funds pandemic preparedness through its Pandemic Fund. That fund is dedicated to "critical investments to strengthen pandemic prevention, preparedness, and response capacities at national, regional, and global levels." The World Bank is especially concerned with investments that aid the pandemic preparedness capacities of low- and middle-income countries. The fund is supported by at least twenty-one donor nations. If that were not enough, the Bill & Melinda Gates Foundation, Wellcome Trust, and the Rockefeller Foundation also contribute to these efforts. Collectively, the Pandemic Fund has $1.6 billion pledged to meet its program goals.

In contrast to public and private investors that focus on pandemic planning, there are a wide range of pandemic response organizations that are on the frontlines fighting disease outbreaks and meeting humanitarian needs wherever they are most needed. It is simply not possible for the governments of this world to respond to a pandemic without recognizing the enormous support provided by an untold number of humanitarian organizations. These organizations, such as the Red Cross, are often asked to provide the resources and staff to meet one or more of the basic needs for food, shelter, and clothing. These services are especially needed for those evicted from their homes, stigmatized by disease, fired from their employment, or refused critical care by overcommitted hospitals and critical care facilities. The Red Cross, one of the oldest humanitarian organizations in the world, has met medical support needs for an untold number of epidemics. Similarly, Doctors without Borders is a non-profit international medical response group that has been on the frontlines combating disease in over seventy nations. Their humanitarian efforts have touched the lives of millions of people. Committed public health and medical workers play a critical role in pandemic response and Doctors without Borders is an organization that plays a central role in protecting public health.

With millions of people infected with disease at any given hour or day of the year, it takes dozens of non-profit organizations and tens of thousands of volunteers and paid staff to meet these medical and humanitarian needs. Another organization that has a track record of responding to public health emergencies is Project Hope. It is an international non-profit organization, with a mission to improve public health around the world. Founded in 1958, Project Hope responds to all kinds of emergencies—not just those associated with infectious disease and pandemics.

The sheer number and variety of pandemic response organizations underscore the challenge of coordinating a coherent international response to novel pathogens. The WHO was established to create consistent policies and procedures to address pandemics. Its efforts remain a work in progress when the world's superpowers have independent pandemic response strategies of their own that may not align with WHO objectives.

## 22. What is disease reporting and why is it important during an epidemic?

Disease that poses a threat to public health is defined as notifiable disease. When such a disease is identified by a physician, private or public health laboratory, or a hospital, immediate reporting to the state public health department is required. There is an expression, "If it isn't measured it isn't managed." This is a management principle that underscores the critical role of accurate data for determining the scope of a public health outbreak. Without adequate reporting it is not possible to calculate the rate of transmission nor the geographic spread of an epidemic disease.

Each state is authorized to establish its own list of notifiable diseases. However, for the benefit of national tracking, the CDC aggregates all the data collected at the county and state levels into a national tracking system. The strength of this system rests on the use of standardized data collection systems using compatible software. However, this remains an ongoing challenge for the CDC. In some cases, data reporting formats, frequency of reporting, data quality, and data transmission formats have jeopardized the timely delivery of critical disease outbreak data.

A general rule of thumb is that disease reporting is never a complete representation of all cases. However, lack of complete reporting does not minimize the value of the data collected. The CDC is able to estimate the scale of an outbreak based on studies that reveal the capture rates of their reporting system. For example, if experience from audits of past reporting initiatives reveals only half of all cases are reported for any given disease, the ability to estimate the scale of an outbreak is fairly easy. Simply multiply reported cases by 2! While this example overs-simplifies the CDC's modelling procedure, it provides a "big picture" perspective on the importance of disease reporting despite its inherent data collection limitations.

The CDC is responsible for the National Notifiable Diseases Surveillance System. This system tracks over seventy separate communicable diseases reported to the CDC from fifty states and territories of the United States. Some key examples of notifiable diseases tracked by the CDC include anthrax, babesiosis, Candida, cholera, cryptosporidiosis, cyclosporiasis, Covid-19, dengue, giardiasis, gonorrhea, hepatitis A, hepatitis, legionellosis, leprosy, listeriosis, malaria, measles, mumps, pneumonia, rabies, rickettsia, Salmonella, salmonellosis, shigellosis, smallpox, tetanus, tuberculosis, typhoid fever, vibriosis, West Nile Fever, yellow fever, and Zika.

Over the period 1992 to 2022, the CDC gradually expanded the number of disease and disease variants tracked from 60 in 1992 to 125 in 2022. The reason for the ever-changing reporting procedures reflects two factors; novel pathogens trigger a focus on enhanced surveillance and therefore disease reporting. Secondly, the rise of variants of disease often requires a special tracking when some mutations become more communicable or lethal than the previously characterized pathogen. Over the last 150 years, notifiable diseases have expanded from a focus on highly communicable diseases—like measles, smallpox, typhoid, and tuberculosis—to less communicable disease like giardiasis and vector-borne disease like Lyme. Over time some diseases have been taken off the list if they no longer pose a threat. However, those added to the list of notifiable diseases are seldom removed. We live in a world of ever-expanding inventories of communicable disease. If a novel pathogen poses a threat to humans, it will be included on the epidemic disease watch list.

## 23. What is contact tracing and how does it reduce the spread of disease?

Contact tracing is the procedure for tracking close contacts of a person infected with a communicable disease. Let's call the infected person, patient zero. The more contacts patient zero has had the greater the challenge posed for public health professionals. Each person who has spent time with patient zero should be tracked down to notify them of their potential exposure. Not everyone who may have been near patient zero is exposed to the disease. For example, in the case of Covid-19, factors that increase risk include (1) the duration of time spent with patient zero; (2) the intensity of the communication, whether, meditating, talking, singing, or shouting; (3) whether patient zero was coughing or sneezing; and (4) whether anyone was wearing face masks during the encounter.

Contact tracing relies on certain assumptions concerning the likelihood of disease transmission in any given instance. Normally, in the case of aerosolized pathogens, the time spent with an individual in close contact in indoor environments will increase the likelihood disease has been transmitted to the susceptible individual. Contact tracing is a critical public health procedure to limit the spread of disease. Those contacted, because of their presumed association with an infected individual, are told to take precautionary measures. These measures include testing, vaccination, isolation, or staying home until it is clear there is no infection. In turn, the secondary contacts of patient zero are also requested to identify the individuals they may have been in contact with. These tertiary level contacts are also notified of their possible exposure to the disease.

In extremely fast-moving epidemics where the time between exposure and infection can be less than four days, infection can spread quickly. In these cases, public health agencies will require dozens of people to serve as contact tracers especially when patient zero had dozens of contacts with other people during his or her infectious period. In many cases, like those experienced with Covid-19, the rapidity with which a disease gets transmitted is influenced by human behavior. For example, in highly congested urban settings such as restaurants, conferences, and sporting events person to person contact is so great the only effective means of tracing these contacts is through cell phone tracking systems.

Cell phone tracking has the advantage of identifying individuals who may not be known to patient zero but happened to be in the same restaurant or conference on that same day and same hour. The disadvantage of cell phone tracking is that it provides no clarity concerning the duration of exposure or the proximity to the individual cell phone holder to patient zero. Cell phone tracking raises many privacy issues that have yet to be resolved. Moreover, there are instances where individuals attending public events do not use cell phones and therefore this method cannot track individuals who are not tied to their phones or who have turned it off.

Contact tracing is normally used to determine the network of potentially infected persons in contact with patient zero. Because each contact with patient zero also has contacts that subsequently occur in various venues, contact tracers must rely on the memory and support of the individuals exposed to patient zero to determine likely third tier exposed individuals. In determining which third tier contacts have been potentially exposed, contact tracers need to know the basic characteristics of the disease. These characteristics include the disease incubation period, its infectious period, the potential for asymptomatic transmission, and the pathogen's ability to survive on fomites including clothing, shared public toilets, tables, and transit systems. These factors may influence which third tier contacts may have been infected.

Each disease has its own unique infectious period—the time during which an exposed individual will become contagious. This information guides contact tracers in identifying the most likely individuals who may be infected. From a practical perspective, contact tracers must take a conservative perspective concerning who merits follow though contact. If a person exposed to patient zero walks home and passes someone on the sidewalk without discussion, will that count as a contact? No, that would be highly unlikely. The basic rule is exposure depends on close contact, long duration and a probable mode of transmission. Aerosolized pathogens can be transmitted over relatively long distances in congested restaurants with poor ventilation systems. At the other extreme, Mpox is transmitted by close physical contact including skin contact and sexual contact. For these reasons contact tracing depends on a basic understanding of the mode of disease transmission and the likelihood any given contact scenario would pose a health risk. Cell phone tracing can't readily achieve these objectives.

Contact tracing is especially valuable when applied in the earliest phases of an outbreak. Its value is drastically reduced when public health agencies have insufficient staff to track fast-moving epidemics. This challenge is made worse when state and local governments have no lockdown or capacity restrictions on places of congregation that harbor disease. Contact tracing works best when there are fewer opportunities for disease transmission. In this context, contact tracing is one of a portfolio of strategies that must work in complement to stop a pandemic. During Covid-19 the rapidity with which disease spread far outstripped government efforts to staff the contact tracing effort. Rather than having one contact tracer for every 1,000 cases, the average staffing was about half that number. Despite the importance of this work, contact tracing was not effective. The situation was like the proverbial Dutch Boy putting his finger in the dam to hold back an impending flood. Without adequate staff in a pandemic scale disease contact tracing only works under strict lockdown, occupancy, and travel restrictions to limit human mobility.

In fast-moving epidemics, lack of contact tracing staff may force public health agencies to prioritize the tracking of individuals posing the greatest risk to vulnerable populations. Those requiring priority protection include nursing homes, assisted living facilities, and the elderly. The Covid-19 pandemic revealed the staffing limitations of American public health agencies. Without adequate staff they were unable to stay abreast when there was an explosion of new cases. This is one of the reasons cell phone tracking concepts were activated; to overcome massive contact tracing staffing shortages. At least twenty-six states tried cell phone applications to track close contacts of infected individuals. One of the primary limitations of these applications was their inability to provide meaningful measurements of distance or exposure—items that are normally addressed by over-the-phone or in-person contact tracing procedures.

State-level cell phone tracing programs were not designed to provide a national perspective on the spread of disease. Each state's contact tracing program operated independently of every other one and therefore interstate carriers of disease were a "lost opportunity." In addition, state programs were only as good as those who choose to participate. One result of limited education and advertising was that many people chose not to participate. Perhaps more importantly, the Government Accounting Office reviewed existing cell phone tracking programs and found problems of trust. Overall Americans are hesitant to turn over personal data to government agencies—even when the purpose of the contact tracing program is well intended and guarantees privacy. Public experience with hacking of government databases over the last twenty years has raised the bar on public acceptance of nice sounding programs without any track record. This is an ongoing impediment to the adoption of cell phone contact tracing programs in America. The rough and tumble effort to try cell phone tracking does not mean it is "dead" forever. Significant investments have been made in the software technology which have not been lost. The future will depend on an even greater investment in education, marketing, and improved proximity resolution software used by two of the major participating organizations—Apple and Google.

## 24. How do vaccines work? How effective are they?

Vaccines work by enhancing our immune system's ability to fight off disease. The purpose of a vaccine is to increase the body's immune response to a specific pathogenic bacterium or virus. Historically, there were two basic ways of achieving this objective. One was by inoculating susceptible individuals with an attenuated form of the virus or bacteria, so the body was not confronted with the pathogen in its full virulence. The other way is to provide a killed version of the virus or bacteria to enable the body's immune response mechanisms to recognize the pathogen without a concern for its virulence or ability to reproduce. Today there are multiple other approaches to make vaccines work including mRNA vaccines like that developed for Covid-19. The use of bioengineered DNA and RNA is now used for a variety of vaccines to stimulate the body's immune system to respond to viable components of bacteria or viruses without its ability to replicate.

The effectiveness of vaccines varies as a result of the body's long-term immune memory for a pathogen. It is not uncommon for some vaccines to require a booster as immunity wanes, or the characteristics of the bacteria or virus change over time. This is true for influenza. The CDC recommends individuals take one dose annually due to the ever-changing characteristics of the influenza virus. Other examples of vaccines that require boosters include the tetanus and diphtheria vaccines. CDC recommends tetanus vaccines be taken every ten years.

The influenza vaccine has always had a relatively low level of effectiveness compared to vaccines designed for measles, mumps, and rubella. Annual vaccination campaigns for influenza provide important protection for many people despite the ongoing challenge of updating the vaccine to current circulating strains. The vaccine's effectiveness is usually under 60 percent and can be as low as 10 percent. The reason for these wide variations in performance is because the vaccine design is based on an anticipated antigen shift in the virus over time. The antigen shift reflects the ongoing variation in the influenza virus strains from one year to the next and this is as much art as it is science.

Recent studies of Covid-19 vaccines—both those based on an mRNA formulation and traditional attenuated virus formulations have shown a high degree of effectiveness in reducing illness and an even higher level of protection from hospitalization. Over time, some of the vaccines have lost their protective value against some strains after six months. This explains the ongoing emphasis on obtaining booster shots to increase immunity to the SARS-CoV-2 infection. The mRNA vaccines created by Moderna and Pfizer were greater than 90 percent effective after six months based on exposure to the original Covid-19 strain. However, with ongoing variants of SARS-CoV-2, their effectiveness waned with the emergence of the Delta variant. Observational studies identified a decreasing effectiveness at four to six months (42–57 percent) for mRNA vaccines against the Delta variant. While the Covid-19 vaccines do not guarantee individuals will not get infected, they play an important role in limiting the severity of disease.

In December 2019, the US FDA approved a vaccine for Ebola. That vaccine relies on a weakened live virus administered as a single dose by injection into a muscle. The weakened live virus contains the vesicular stomatitis virus altered to contain a gene from the Ebola virus. A study of this vaccine found it to be 100 percent effective against Ebola. For those with vaccine hesitancy the proposition is quite simple; in a hypothetical Ebola outbreak in your neighborhood would you prefer to take your chances without the protection offered by the vaccine hoping your immune system would save the day? Or would you prefer to take a vaccine that is 100 percent effective and deal with possible adverse side effects that might not be known at this time? That is the classic dilemma we all face in a world of risk management. What choice would you make? Obviously, the decision would depend on our perception of the risk and the likelihood we might become infected.

Similarly, the CDC has found the three types of human papillomavirus vaccines to be extremely effective in reducing HPV infections. However, only one of these vaccines is available in the United States—Gardasil-9. The greater challenge remains improving public awareness and use of the approved HPV vaccines. The HPV vaccines are a remarkable achievement. For many years HPV was a cancer without cure. It took many years for this cancer to be recognized as caused by a virus. These vaccines are an important tool in efforts to reduce sexually transmitted disease.

Two doses of the Measles, Mumps, and Rubella (MMR) vaccine are 97 percent effective in preventing these diseases. The measles vaccination program started in 1963. At that time an estimated 3 to 4 million Americans got measles each year. Since then, the measles virus-containing vaccine has led to a greater than 99 percent reduction in measles cases compared with the pre-vaccine era. It is important to note, measles is still common in other countries operating with inadequate health care systems, limited access to vaccines and with malnourished and poverty-stricken populations.

The diphtheria, tetanus, and whooping cough vaccine is 97 percent effective for a ten-year period. CDC has authorized nine recombinant vaccines which not only provide protection for these three diseases but also protect against other diseases as well. Some of the recombinant vaccines address Haemophilus influenzae type b disease, hepatitis B, and polio. The level of protection against diphtheria, tetanus, and whooping cough decreases with time and for this reason ten-year boosters are recommended. Diphtheria was once a major cause of illness and death among children in the United States. In 1921, 206,000 cases of diphtheria were recorded in the United States causing 15,520 deaths. With the introduction of vaccination, diphtheria rates dropped quickly in the United States as well as in other countries. Because of the success of the US vaccination program, diphtheria is a rare disease in the United States. In contrast, more than

22,900 cases were reported to the WHO in 2019, but many more cases are simply not reported.

Cholera has long been the cause of many epidemics around the world. There are numerous oral vaccines available to prevent cholera and the effectiveness of these vaccines varies. One study conducted of a two-dose oral vaccine found a 79 percent effectiveness during a cholera epidemic in Zanzibar during the years 2009–10. That study also noted immunization efforts not only protected individuals but also provided herd immunity benefits for unvaccinated members of the community who came into contact with those who took the oral vaccine.

## 25. How do researchers create vaccines for new diseases?

Medical researchers start by identifying the pathogen for which a vaccine is needed. This is not always easy for novel pathogens where little is known about their characteristics. In many instances there may be numerous variants of a pathogen so it may be important to decide if the vaccine is intended to address one specific variant or if the effort will be to develop a more universal vaccine to address numerous variants of the pathogen of concern. On a broader level researchers also must consider five criteria before developing a vaccine. The vaccine must (1) be able to protect against the disease for which it is intended, (2) be safe and not have any adverse health effects, (3) provide long-term protection, (4) create antibodies that can neutralize the antigens included in the vaccine, and (5) be practical by being relatively stable in various temperature regimes and easily administered.

Researchers must decide whether to use a whole killed vaccine or focus on subunits of the pathogen that are more appropriate for developing an immune response. Alternatively, an attenuated organism can be used for a vaccine—one that has lost its virulence but remains alive. However, attenuated organisms can pose risks if the attenuated organism reverts back to its virulent state. Yet live organisms generally provide a stronger immune response than killed organisms. The vaccine for MMR uses an attenuated organism. This is also true for the polio vaccine.

The third option is creating what is called a recombinant DNA vaccine by inserting the genes for specific antigens into the genomes of non-virulent organisms. The antigens are various substances such as toxins, components of bacteria, or viruses that when introduced into the human body stimulate the production of antibodies. A fourth type of vaccine is called a non-replicating viral vector vaccine. These vaccines do not reproduce at all. They are developed using a harmless carrier virus that has an inserted gene encoded for the antigen of the pathogen of concern. Upon being exposed to the vaccine the body will react to create antibodies. That activates the immune system. The adenovirus is one of the common viral vectors used for the development of this type of vaccine. A fifth type of vaccine approach is the virus-like particle vaccine. This approach assembles multiple copies of structural proteins found in infectious virus particles. However, these particles do not contain genetic material but provide an important activation function for the body's surveillance cells—a key aspect of the immune system. This is a non-living vaccine and for this reason an adjuvant is required. An adjuvant is a non-toxic, biodegradable material intended to enhance the immunological response of the body to the vaccine.

Finally, since the development of the Covid-19 mRNA vaccines, a vaccine may be developed using the messenger RNA method by inserting the antigen into the structure of a bioengineered RNA agent. The antigen is selected for which the body will develop a strong antibody response. The mRNA vaccine when injected into the body uses the recipient's own cells to produce the encoded proteins. The mRNA vaccines have not necessarily lived up to the fourth criteria of an effective vaccine—their effective response has waned because of the ever-changing variants of SARS-CoV-2. Nevertheless, the mRNA vaccines represent a major step forward in the development of new delivery systems for generating an immune response in the human body. It also represents the first time in history that a vaccine has been created to respond to a pandemic in progress. In this sense, the mRNA vaccine is one of the greatest achievements in the field of vaccine research.

## 26. What non-pharmaceutical measures work to combat epidemics when effective vaccines or antibiotics don't exist?

There are a wide range of non-pharmaceutical measures used when vaccines or antibiotics do not exist or are unavailable for immediate use. The specific measures taken depend on the mode of transmission of the disease and the degree to which it has taken hold within a community, state, or nation. Respiratory diseases are perhaps of the greatest concern since they can be communicated without close contact with other people. The measures available can be divided into two basic categories: those appropriate for individual action and those that must be initiated at the governmental level.

Individuals can protect themselves from respiratory disease by minimizing close contact with other people in indoor settings, wearing a face mask when in close contact with others, and avoiding crowded indoor events. One could become a monk and isolate in a remote monastery, but such a practice might not be possible for those that hold steady jobs in the work world. For this reason, personal risk management depends on recognizing how to navigate the various risks that come with buying groceries, spending time in theaters, attending church, riding on a train, bus, or airplane, and attending school. In each of these scenarios, absent governmental orders concerning human behavior, each person must consider how to minimize risk in these potentially pathogen exposing scenarios.

At the governmental level, when an outbreak or epidemic is recognized, the first and most important non-pharmaceutical measure to undertake is to provide information on the nature of the disease. This must include how it is transmitted and the risks it poses to human health. Public health education is the first and most critical element of any non-pharmaceutical intervention. Public education prepares the ground for public understanding of proper personal behavior and responsibility for one's behavior as it affects others. Risk communication is an essential part of this first phase of a governmental response. At a minimum, it requires individuals with expertise in risk communication as well as knowledge of the nature of disease transmission. The portfolio of interventions that may be activated depends on the nature, spread, and location of the epidemic. When a disease has been identified within a school system, the logical focus will be on school closure, remote schooling, or a hybrid teaching approach using remote teaching with in-school measures such as face masks and social distancing. The options selected depend on a thorough investigation of the sources and means of transmission. If the disease has passed from the children to family members, it may be necessary to require those exposed to stay home and isolate from other members of the family.

However, if the epidemic has gone well beyond the school system, and to the parents and siblings of the infected children, then further lockdowns may be required. Lockdowns is a recently coined term to describe the closure of public or private buildings that may serve as points of transmission for disease. Closing places of congregation is an option that works but also comes with a significant economic cost to the businesses affected. Closing businesses also affects the life of citizens who depend on their services. The consequences of lockdowns can be disastrous for theaters, restaurants, gymnasiums, coffee houses, and other places of congregation where people meet for social, sustenance, and recreational needs. An alternative approach, adopted by some states during Covid-19, included limiting maximum indoor seating capacities, requiring greater separations between users of restaurants, gymnasiums, theaters, etc., and requiring face masks for those entering indoor environments (see question 29).

Furthermore, routine sanitation and disinfection may be required for places where people routinely congregate. These measures can lessen the transmission of disease caused by hand to mouth behavior. These behavioral and sanitation measures may also be combined with engineering controls. For example, improved building heating, cooling and ventilating systems, can serve as substitutes for the more draconian closure of businesses during a pandemic. There is extensive evidence that poor air circulation in restaurants, bars, gymnasiums, and theaters contributed to the spread of Covid-19.

Non-pharmaceutical interventions that can be of great value often take time to develop and implement. For example, schools, restaurants, and other places of congregation can dramatically reduce airborne pathogens by installing ventilation systems. A well-designed vent system can increase the number of air changes per hour and that in turn lessens the concentration of airborne pathogens within the building. In addition, some facilities including hospitals and nursing homes should consider installing ultraviolet light disinfection systems within the air ducts. A building disinfection system reduces pathogen exposure by not re-entraining contaminated air back into the occupied space. Moreover, because high rates of air changes per hour also result in increased costs for heating in the winter months, air to air heat exchangers are recommended. Air to air heat exchangers capture the warmth from the air to be expelled to the outside without losing its heat. Such innovations can play a significant role in reducing exposure to disease but often take time and money. Moreover, these types of engineering controls are unlikely to be a priority during an epidemic. Improvements to building ventilation systems often are the outcome of the lessons learned from a past epidemic. One interim measure, adopted during the Covid-19 epidemic, was offering outdoor dining, opening windows inside restaurants, and providing fans. Depending upon how these short-term fixes are installed, they may help minimize person to person exposure to airborne pathogens.

For diseases transmitted through food or water the countermeasures will be dramatically different than for aerosol transmitted disease. State public health regulations have detailed procedures for improving the sanitary conditions in restaurants and other establishments serving food or beverages. However, state public health regulations do not govern the sanitary conditions in the home. Each of us must become familiar with the dangers posed by eating food that has not been cleaned or cooked.

Because of potential bioterrorist threats to public drinking water supplies, water companies have developed security plans to protect water quality and increase the monitoring of water supply reservoirs and aquifer protection zones. These non-pharmaceutical strategies reflect a growing awareness that waterborne disease could easily be transmitted to millions of innocent people by the actions of rogue actors. Dumping large quantities of *Vibrio cholerae* or similar pathogens into a public water supply could create a public health disaster for any municipal water supply in America. Protecting our nation's water supplies from such potential threats is an example of a non-pharmaceutical measure to prevent an epidemic—rather than combating one that slipped through the reservoir's security system.

## 27. What is the difference between quarantine and isolation? How do they help combat epidemics?

Quarantine is designed to sequester individuals who were exposed to a disease whereas isolation is designed to confine individuals who have been infected with disease. This distinction is a modern one developed by physicians of the nineteenth century to avoid using the term quarantine for those placed in hospital settings. In the nineteenth-century America, the term quarantine conjured visions of being exiled to offshore islands where limited medical support was available and the chances of recovery from disease were not favorable. Physicians of the nineteenth century, particularly those in the Boston area where the concept of isolation hospitals was first developed, envisioned a hospital that would provide adequate air, ventilation, and care for those with an infectious disease. This was a major step forward in a more humane treatment of those with a contagious disease. Prior to the development of isolation hospitals, it was not uncommon for everyone to be placed in one shared quarantine facility—even when only one person was infected. It didn't matter whether you were infected or not—all residents of a specific building were quarantined together. Quarantine, despite its important role in slowing disease transmission, was feared by the public. Confinement was not a voluntary choice. In reaction to past applications of quarantine, a modernized approach was adopted by the American Public Health Association (APHA) in 1917. It formed the basis for state-level quarantine regulations that exist today. The 1917 APHA definitions recognized the difference between those infected and those exposed to a communicable disease. Initially clinical symptoms of disease were used to identify the infected but over time this evolved into the use of various testing regimens able to identify infection through genetic or antigen-specific testing procedures.

The purpose of quarantine is to stop the unintended transmission of a communicable disease by someone who may be exposed and may soon become infectious. Quarantine stops the spread of disease if the period of quarantine is sufficient to cover the period during which that individual is infectious— meaning capable of spreading the disease to others. Quarantines have historically been supervised by public health or medical staff to ensure individuals adhered to their confinement. In these circumstances, those quarantined were provided with adequate food and care. In addition, guards were often assigned to quarantined houses to be sure those confined inside did not go out shopping or slip away from their confinement. The fiscal resources to fund guards at each quarantined house were inevitably inadequate especially in large-scale epidemics. One solution used in the past was the installation of temporary outdoor tents where the infected could be treated as a group thereby reducing overhead costs for guards and other support staff.

In modern times, as witnessed with Covid-19, the lack of public health or medical staff and the rapidity with which virus was transmitted made voluntary quarantines the new paradigm. It was simply the only option in a situation where millions were infected and tens of millions were exposed. While the effectiveness of quarantine might not have been perfect based on an honor system, it was the best available means to protect the affected community. Individuals in a voluntary quarantine scenario are expected to minimize human contact until they have exceeded the incubation period for the disease. If after quarantine the individual is without symptoms they are released, otherwise they are isolated.

Isolation is required until the symptoms disappear, and the patient is no longer infectious. When resources exist, isolation would normally take place in a hospital setting but this may not always be possible when an entire community is besieged with hundreds of similar cases (see question 39). In such instances, the help of visiting nurses or other support staff may be required to provide care for the individual in their own residence or other emergency medical setting. In other instances, even that level of support may be unavailable if there are insufficient public health staff and fiscal resources. As a last resort, those in isolation or quarantine may only get public health support through phone calls, zoom meetings, and/or email. In effect the level and type of support provided for those in quarantine or isolation must be scalable to work within the public health resources available.

Triage becomes the operative term when epidemics burn out the resources needed to control them. When public health resources are insufficient to combat an epidemic, the resources that exist must be parsed out so the most good can be done at the least cost. If the goal is saving lives, then the focus must be on the most vulnerable who are most easily treated or protected. However, if the goal is to stop the epidemic as quickly as possible then scarce resources may be better focused on contact tracing to break the chain of transmission. These are the life and death choices that must be made when vaccines or antibiotic treatments are not available, or an insufficient supply exists to meet demand.

## 28.  What are universal public health precautions?

The CDC developed the concept of universal health precautions for hospitals. Within a hospital setting these precautions include (1) wearing gloves and gowns if there is soiling of hands, exposed skin, or clothing with blood or body fluids likely; (2) wearing a mask and protective eyewear or chin length plastic face shields whenever splashing or splattering of blood or other body fluids could occur; (3) washing hands before and after any contact with patients and after removal of gloves including replacing gloves between each patient visit; (4) using a disposable mouthpiece for cardiopulmonary resuscitation; (5) immediately disposing of contaminated needles into a puncture proof container without bending, pinching, or clipping needles during disposal; and (6) cleaning spills of blood or contaminated body fluids by putting on gloves and other necessary barriers and wiping up with disposable towels. This measure also requires washing with soap and water and then disinfecting with a 1:10 solution of household bleach and water. The solution should be set for at least 10 minutes and should be made within 24 hours of its use. These universal precautions apply to hospital settings but may be valuable for other settings where medical or occupational health personnel work with similar concerns for sanitation.

However, the concept of universal health precautions goes far beyond procedures unique to hospital transmission of disease. Universal health precautions are principles that recognize the multi-faceted ways in which communicable disease can be transmitted between people and vectors of disease. If everyone on the planet were to practice basic precautionary principles disease transmission could be dramatically reduced. These precautions include (1) hand-washing before meals; (2) adopting cough etiquette—covering your mouth when you sneeze; (3) applying insect repellent or wearing mosquito proof clothing when outdoors during mosquito season; (4) properly cleaning and cooking food before consumption; (5) boiling water before use if relying on river, lake, or spring water for consumption; (6) avoiding the use of common eating utensils; (7) routinely cleaning and disinfecting common kitchen and bathroom surfaces used by multiple users; (8) wearing a tightly fit face mask around persons who are sick; (9) vaccinating children as recommended by the CDC childhood immunization schedule; and (10) staying home when sick. Adoption of these universal health precautions requires the support of local, state, and federal public health agencies, the public-school systems, and the parents of all children on the planet. Individual human behavior matters and these precautions play an important role in limiting disease transmission. Personal health responsibilities are our responsibility. Yet they also contribute to the public health of our community. We are all connected by the germs that surround us.

Mosquito-borne disease such as Zika, yellow fever, malaria, and dengue can be avoided by wearing mosquito proof clothes, using insect repellent, and making sure window screens are properly functioning throughout the home. Similarly, exposure to cholera, Salmonella, and giardia can be avoided by adopting food cleaning, water sanitation practices, and boiling water whenever relying on river or spring water on camping trips. Perhaps the most valuable precautions are those that minimize our exposure to airborne disease like SARS, Influenza, and Covid-19. Adopting cough etiquette, wearing face masks during epidemics, and staying home when sick all help reduce the likelihood of disease transmission. Finally, a great deal can be done to contain communicable disease simply by getting vaccinated and making sure our children are also vaccinated following the childhood immunization schedule. That immunization schedule calls for childhood vaccinations for (1) hepatitis B; (2) diphtheria, tetanus, and pertussis; (3) polio; (4) MMR; (5) varicella; (6) influenza; and (7) *Haemophilus influenzae* type b.

## 29. Do public health mandates to control human behavior work?

The success of any public health mandate depends on the degree to which the public has been informed of the benefits of any given mandate for both the individual and the broader community. Public acceptance also depends on the duration and severity of the impacts as weighed against the benefits achieved. For example, if a state public health director orders the closure of schools in a city due to a measles outbreak but fails to provide an explanation for this action or fails to mention the length of the school closure or the criteria for reviewing this decision, parents and teachers may react quite negatively. To make a mandate acceptable in a democratic society the affected stakeholders must be engaged in the decision-making process. A mandate issued without any details or even a brief opportunity for public input, guarantees the mandate will be poorly received.

The expertise and communication skills of public health or medical experts play an important role in guiding acceptance of public health mandates. Throughout American history there have been examples where quarantine was imposed quite successfully. In these cases, both the public, the business community and the medical profession recognized the need for mandatory restrictions on human behavior in the interest of the general health, safety, and welfare of the community. Similarly, there have been numerous examples of just the opposite scenarios; public rebellion against the imposition of quarantine measures when done through unilateral decisions made by elected leaders. Lacking a participatory process to engage the people affected by quarantines, it should be no surprise affected citizens will react negatively.

We live in a society with hundreds of recommendations and mandates which we follow on a routine basis. For example, Americans by and large (1) stop at red lights on busy intersections; (2) annually pay their local, state, and federal taxes; (3) vaccinate their children for the recommended immunizations established by the CDC; (4) avoid crossing urban streets until the walk sign lights up, and dozens of other socially accepted forms of behavior. In this context, when a public health order is issued, its success will depend on its social acceptance. Social acceptance is influenced by peer pressure. In this context, key influencers play an outsize role in establishing the legitimacy of any given mandate. Doctors and public health professionals are thought leaders and influence human behavior. However even these individuals must develop risk communication skills if they wish to be effective leaders in the midst of an epidemic. They must become the pied pipers who charm the public with their oratory, charisma, and expertise to follow their lead. This is a tall order in a society where many people question authority.

The advantage of a socially accepted public health mandate is that public health behaviors represent a "we" approach—not a "you do what we tell you approach." This is a significant difference between successful public health mandates and those that fail miserably. One way to achieve the desired "socially acceptable" mandate is for public health professionals to provide choices concerning public health strategies to achieve the desired goal. The public is thereby given a choice in the process. This approach means evaluating the benefits and risks of each option, so a decision carries the weight of a public process into the final decision. The psychology of turning a public health mandate into a public consensus is a critical component of the process. Government of the people, for the people, and by the people is the ideal. However, it is important to bear in mind as our nation has gotten larger, with multiple layers of government and with limited individual involvement in decision making at higher levels of government, participatory decision-making is harder to achieve. A practical solution is to have a large bull horn to reach the ears of everybody in town. In the modern world that would be access to a sympathetic media. We inevitably must rely on the role of the media to persuade various interest groups of the benefits of measures to stop an epidemic. It may not always be easy to muster the support of the media—whether that be television talk show hosts, newspaper editors, radio station commentators, or blogsites on the internet. In a society with literally thousands of self-proclaimed reporters and commentators critiquing government decision-making, the public will search for credible sources of information to verify the costs and benefits of public health orders. Therein lies the challenge we face in the twenty-first century.

Those charged with initiating unpopular public health mandates such as lockdowns, school closures, community level quarantines, or required use of face masks in public settings must be experts and they must be ready for their "A" game. These include mustering technical support staff to back up their recommendations with convincing evidence for the best path forward. Public health measures of nationwide consequence require the expertise of more than one individual. A team approach is necessary for highly complex emergencies that impact human behavior, the economy, public health, and the emotional well-being of an entire society. This has often been the biggest failure found in past public health mandates; not all the experts were brought to bear on the wide range of secondary impacts created by mandates that closed the nation's public schools. In complex emergencies dozens of experts are needed to address every aspect of human behavior, legal requirements, technological, economic, and cultural considerations. Government actions may have unintended consequences and this must be understood and addressed in any pandemic response plan. The days of "solo playing," where one person pretends to have all the answers, are long gone.

The earlier public consensus is achieved during an epidemic the greater our ability to stop its spread. In the nineteenth century, epidemic disease was routine and public acceptance of public health mandates, while not universal, was less controversial than it has been during the twenty-first century. The challenge of the twenty-first century is developing public education programs and infrastructure capable of mobilizing resources at the outset of an outbreak. Practice makes perfect and America's preparedness planning still has a long way to go. Preparedness planning is a tall order in a society with an inadequate investment in basic public health services, medical research, and hospital capacity in an age of pandemics. Getting consensus at the start of an epidemic is much like a shotgun wedding. The unwilling couple has no interest in the marriage contract and the minister is not too convincing about the sacred vows. That is why pandemic planning that begins the day after the epidemic is announced is too little too late.

## 30. Covid-19 revealed political differences in the way pandemics are managed. Is this a new phenomenon?

Political differences concerning the way epidemics or pandemics are managed is not a new phenomenon. Throughout American history the party in power during an epidemic has taken criticism for failing to stop the spread of disease in a timely manner. For example, the city of Boston's response to the 1871 to 1873 smallpox epidemic was a classic example of a failure of political leadership. Public opposition to the "do nothing" politicians was so great that two-thirds of the Boston City Council were voted out of office during the height of the epidemic. Indeed, despite a belated effort by the city council—composed of a common council and a board of aldermen—to establish an independent board of health on December 2, 1872, the public considered their efforts "too little and too late." The "do nothing" city council members along with Boston mayor William Gaston were voted out of office on December 10. It didn't matter that the city council had created a professional board of health ten days earlier. That paled into insignificance compared to the previous twelve months of blame shifting, foot dragging, and political ineptitude. This was a major setback for William Gaston, the democratic mayor of Boston. Gaston championed public health reforms but was unable to move the cumbersome machinery of Boston politics in a timely manner. In part the cause of his loss was due to the overly complicated decision-making process of Boston's bi-cameral form of government. It also reflected the city's failure to establish an independent board of health run by professionals—not by Boston's ward politicians. He lost a close election to Henry L. Pierce simply because the city had politicized virtually every aspect of public health decision-making (Vidich, 2020).

The yellow fever epidemics of the 1790s was the first national example of a political divide in dealing with communicable disease. Yellow fever was entering American port cities including, Philadelphia, Boston, and New York during the summer months. No one was quite sure how yellow fever was transmitted and the result was the political parties of that era had differing strategies for its control. Those who believed it was caused by miasmas blamed the problem on foul air coming from rotting food wastes, swamp gas, dead animals, and open sewers. This faction advocated for improved sanitation controls. In contrast, those who believed the disease was contagious and was brought into American ports by ships coming from the tropics advocated for quarantine. The battle between these competing disease theories was carried out during the last two years of George Washington's presidency. For those concerned with the impact of yellow fever on business, quarantine was viewed as an impediment to trade. The political stakes were high because the federal government at that time did not have quarantine authority; that was the exclusive prerogative of the states. Many congressmen feared expanding the authority of the fledgling federal government into the domain of public health. Despite their worst fears, many other congressmen, particularly those in the Southern states, called for change. They realized epidemics could not be stopped by the individual efforts of states working in isolation from their neighbors. The Fourth Congress of the United States that spanned the period March 4, 1795, to March 4, 1797, made public health a federal prerogative that complemented the public health authorities of the states by creating national oversight over epidemics. This was the first American political debate about epidemic disease in Congress and, while it became the law of the land, it was not unanimously supported by the political parties of that era (see question 5).

For every major epidemic and pandemic in American history, there have almost always been political conflicts on their management. Public health and humanitarian efforts undertaken during epidemics were debated at every level of government especially the local level. In the colonial era epidemics were primarily managed by cities and towns with some guidance provided by colonial governments. Conflicts with the business interests in American port cities were inevitable whenever an epidemic struck Boston. Imagine a major American city locked down for several weeks or months without access to essential goods or services. Cities like Boston lived and died on their access to the vital network of trade routes and farms and cottage industries in the hinterland. Caught between the adverse consequences of maritime quarantines and restricted access to country trade, merchants like John Hancock declared their business suffered terribly. These business impacts played out in the political arena of early American town meetings where decisions were made (Vidich, 2020).

Indeed, there is a rich literature on this topic particularly in the case of untold numbers of bungled quarantine strategies associated with efforts to stop smallpox, cholera, yellow fever, and typhoid outbreaks. These bungled efforts were the catalyst for the creation of local and state-level public health departments across the United States. Under public pressure, mob violence and significant loss of life, the divisive politics of epidemics led to intense calls for government reform. Amid crisis divided political parties knelt before public demands for professional approaches to controlling epidemics. Epidemics were the catalysts that created America's public health system.

# Protecting Yourself during an
# Epidemic or Pandemic

## 31. Will past exposure to an epidemic disease protect against future exposures to that disease?

The answer is it depends on whether the disease has mutated since an individual's past exposure and the degree of exposure that individual may have had. Some diseases, like smallpox, provided a lifetime immunity for those infected. In contrast, a previous infection with influenza does not guarantee exposure to a subsequent strain will be protective against infection. Similarly, those infected by dengue may be protected from the strain with which they were infected but that may not provide protection to three other strains of the dengue virus.

Is a greater immunity achieved by prior infection to a communicable disease when one is fortunate enough to recover or will a vaccine provide longer protection? While this is an academic question for those interested in avoiding disease, it has some relevance for those previously infected and pondering the benefit of a vaccine during the onset of a second epidemic. There is no evidence of the effectiveness of gaining immunity through infection versus through a vaccine-induced immunity. However, the purpose of vaccines is to prevent disease and to the extent that approved vaccines exist, they will always be a better choice than accidental or purposeful infection from a communicable disease.

The World Health Organization (WHO) has identified twenty-six diseases where vaccines provide protection from future exposures. These diseases are cholera; COVID-19; dengue; diphtheria; hepatitis; *Haemophilus influenzae* type b (Hib); human papillomavirus (HPV); influenza; Japanese encephalitis; malaria; measles; meningococcal meningitis; mumps; pertussis; pneumococcal disease; poliomyelitis; rabies; rotavirus; rubella; tetanus; tick-borne encephalitis; tuberculosis; typhoid; varicella; and yellow fever. The annual influenza vaccines provide some protection from any given strain of influenza circulating in any given area of the world. In May 2022, the WHO found vaccine effectiveness ranged from 59 percent to 77 percent depending on the type of vaccine formulation for those eighteen to sixty-five years of age. These vaccine efficacy results are somewhat more promising than those reported by the Centers for Disease Control and Prevention (CDC). Overall, the level of protection and the length of immunity offered by vaccines varies widely.

Rather than speculating on the relative immunity created by past exposure, the best course of action should always be to get a booster when an epidemic is imminent. A 2007 *New England Journal of Medicine* study found infection or vaccination for measles, mumps, rubella, and varicella provided the equivalent of lifetime protection. In contrast, tetanus vaccinations require boosters about every ten years and diphtheria vaccinations—when offered as a disease-specific vaccine—were only good for about nineteen years. These findings also note diphtheria-tetanus vaccine has a different impact on antibodies than those vaccines designed for one disease only. Prior infection to a disease provides a degree of immunity for some time but the length of that protection varies widely depending on the disease. At one extreme, vaccines for influenza are the least protective over time due to the ever-changing strains found in any given geographic area of the world. In contrast, infection or exposure to measles, mumps, and rubella provide a very long-lasting protection against future exposures.

Past exposure to cholera provides long-lasting immunity to specific serogroups of that disease. Organisms with similar antigens are considered a serogroup. There are two strains of cholera, referred to as serogroups 01 and 0139. Infection from cholera serogroup 01 does not provide immunity to serogroup 0139. Fortunately, there is now an oral cholera vaccine that is quite effective against serogroup 01. The WHO Global Task Force on Cholera Control (GTFCC) is committed to reducing cholera by 90 percent by the year 2030 in most of the cholera infected nations.

While prior exposure to well-known and well-studied pathogens has given us a good handle on immunity induced through infection, all bets are off when the world faces a novel pathogen. If you should get infected by a novel pathogen like SARSs-Covid-2, we now know complete immunity is fleeting. Novel pathogens, by definition, pose the greatest threat to human health since there are no vaccines to come to the rescue. Without past exposure to a novel pathogen, we play a game of Russian Roulette where humans have the distinct disadvantage of playing with a loaded gun.

## 32.  What personal choices influence exposure to disease?

Personal choice depends on one's health education. Start by learning about the risks posed by prevalent communicable disease in your geographic region. Then make choices founded on evidence. Those not familiar with disease prevalent nearby are not likely to be prepared. Right understanding leads to right action. Personal choice starts with dramatic improvements in our collective understanding of communicable disease in general and those that have the potential to trigger epidemics in particular.

Personal choice, at a fundamental level, means getting enough regular exercise, sufficient sleep and a proper diet. These personal choices do not protect us from exposure to an epidemic disease. However, they increase our chance of fighting it off. Stress, lack of sleep, lack of exercise, and a poor diet are factors adversely affecting our immune system. For example, those suffering from obesity, diabetes, and chronic obstructive pulmonary disease are more vulnerable to communicable disease than those who are in good health. Good health starts with a good education in personal hygiene that gradually leads to better decisions in the mental, emotional, and physical arenas of our lives. Right understanding leads to right action and our personal choices are strongly influenced by the public health values of the society in which we live.

A third factor influencing our personal health is the company we keep. When we hang around those who smoke, consume alcohol, or take recreational drugs we are far more likely to be influenced by peer pressure and take up one or more of these habits. While it may not always be possible to avoid environments where alcohol is served, smoking is permitted and recreational drugs are taken, we should never forget that our own health depends on our personal choices. None of these three habits are good for our health. America is facing an "epidemic" level of recreational drug use that has resulted in hundreds of thousands of annual deaths. In 2020, the CDC reported 91,799 drug overdose deaths took place in the United States. The National Institute of Health reports an estimated 95,000 Americans die from alcohol-related causes annually. Cigarette smoking remains the leading cause of preventable disease, disability, and death in the United States, accounting for more than 480,000 deaths a year, or about one in five deaths. Combined drugs, alcohol, and smoking cause an estimated 666,799 deaths annually. All of these are preventable through personal choice. These habits compromise our immune system making it that much harder to fight off exposure to highly lethal pathogens.

Personal choice also comes into play at the outset of an outbreak or epidemic. The choices we make during a crisis pose a greater risk if (1) we fail to become disease savvy and (2) fail to consult with public health and medical experts concerning appropriate personal behavior during an epidemic. However, personal choice is not limited to epidemic conditions alone. Our choices during non-epidemic conditions also matter. Personal choices that make a huge difference include getting vaccinated against (1) mumps, measles, and rubella; (2) the human papillomavirus for sexually active individuals; and (3) cholera and yellow fever when traveling to overseas destinations where these diseases are endemic (see question 33). Personal choice means adopting sanitary procedures for cooking and cleaning of food, maintaining a healthy lifestyle, and practicing safe sex (see question 36).

## 33.  What are the most effective ways to protect oneself when an epidemic or pandemic occurs?

Become informed of the public health risks posed by an epidemic disease. Adopt personal behavior that avoids exposure to people and places most likely to harbor disease. And encourage your friends and family to follow these practices. In many cases, an epidemic or pandemic involves the appearance of a novel pathogen for which there are no vaccines. In the case of epidemics involving a known pathogen, vaccines should be first line of protection. However, even if a vaccine exists, there may be an inadequate supply to address the immediate demand. Pandemics are rarely stopped through approved vaccines. For one, pandemic disease often represents either a novel pathogen or a known pathogen that has mutated enough to render existing vaccines useless. This is particularly true for the seasonal influenza virus that changes from year to year. Influenza vaccines may provide some benefit but there is no guarantee. Vaccine development is a year-long process and the strain for which the vaccine is created may turn out to be different than anticipated by the vaccine manufacturer.

It is a highly unlikely scenario to find an adequate supply of vaccine available at the outset of an epidemic. Yet a vaccine protected population is the ultimate goal. Achieving this goal establishes herd immunity which in turn stops the spread of disease. However, it is the diseases for which vaccines do not exist that pose the greatest threat. Given this predicament, the emphasis must be on other forms of personal and community level protection that rely on non-pharmaceutical interventions (see question 26). Just as we have seen with Covid-19, vaccines took close to a year to be developed. It took even longer to achieve a high level of vaccine penetration within America and even longer elsewhere in the world. Indeed, many nations are still woefully under-vaccinated simply because the wealthier nations assigned highest priority to distribution of vaccines to their own people. In almost all past epidemics and pandemics, personal and community-sanctioned behaviors made a difference in whether a pathogen spread or died out. Last minute edicts to control human behavior generally are a sour pill. Americans are used to freedom of mobility, freedom of speech, and freedom of choice. The key to effective personal protection rests on being fully informed from credible sources about the risks posed by exposure to epidemic-scale pathogens.

Similarly, experts must become more familiar with the psychology of communication and the science of influence. Learning about safe personal behaviors is more effective when we take the advice to heart. When we perceive suggestions as edicts from government bureaucrats, we take offense. A common reaction is to dismiss edicts especially when issued by someone unfamiliar with our predicament in life. With very few exceptions, the science and art of influence has been one of the greatest skills lacking amongst medical, public health, and political leaders in charge of stopping epidemics. This has been the history of the last two hundred years. Developing the skills of the Pied Piper, the man who led the rats out of a plague infested German city, is an example of the charm it takes to move people's heart through compassion and not fear.

There is no such thing as a generic epidemic or pandemic response plan. Yet the threats posed by disease that have the potential to become epidemic have three things in common; they have a high basic reproductive number, a high case fatality rate, and a short incubation period. Epidemic diseases that fit these criteria include, cholera, Covid-19, diphtheria, measles, monkey pox, pneumonic plague, rubella, SARS, and scarlet fever. While tuberculosis does not have a short incubation period it is one of the most dangerous pandemic capable diseases. All these diseases are ones for which quarantine and isolation procedures have been developed to respond to disease outbreaks.

Since some epidemic disease may be transmitted as a droplet or an aerosol, limiting exposure to these diseases is quite challenging. In contrast, when transmission is caused by ingestion of food contaminated with Salmonella, cholera, or typhoid, exposure control depends on careful attention to food and water sanitation. Specific measures to protect oneself include proper disinfection of food preparation areas, bathroom fixtures, and commonly used cutlery, silverware, and other food preparation equipment. Contamination by small quantities of these pathogens can be the first step in the natural evolution of an epidemic.

These examples underscore the importance of public education as the first and fundamental step in protecting oneself from epidemic scale disease. Starting the educational program, the day after an outbreak is already too late to engage the rational mind. Success requires a culture-wide long-term engagement within the American educational system. It should start in grade school and must progress through the American higher education system if we expect to create a culture of public health. Practice makes perfect. The more we prepare for outbreaks the better we will be at protecting ourselves when the big one comes.

## 34. Is handwashing effective for reducing exposure to epidemic diseases?

Handwashing is an important public health measure especially for foodborne and waterborne disease. To a lesser extent, it is also an important strategy in avoiding airborne and vector-borne disease. In 2006, the CDC identified thirty-one pathogens that caused foodborne illness in the United States. During that year an estimated 9.4 million Americans were sickened by eating contaminated food. While not all these cases are associated with an epidemic, the sheer number of foodborne diseases underscores the importance of handwashing. What makes handwashing so important is that 80 percent of all infectious diseases are transmitted by touch (Philip M. Tierno, Secret Life of Germs, 2001). Infectious diseases that rely on touch to infect us include the common cold, the highly lethal Ebola virus, monkeypox, and numerous foodborne and waterborne diseases like cholera and Salmonella.

Unfortunately, very few Americans practice handwashing. A study conducted in Grand Central station public bathrooms in New York City found over 60 percent of all bathroom users failed to wash their hands. Indeed, fewer than 10 percent of the bathroom users washed their hands to an adequate level. These are not unusual findings. Viruses and bacteria are invisible to the naked eye and therefore human behavior is not influenced by things that can't be seen.

Yet handwashing is only one of several protective measures to avoid contact with disease causing organisms. Hand to mouth transmission of disease is common. However, disease can also be transmitted by contaminated food and in such instances, handwashing is only one of many required protective measures. For example, it is important to adopt proper cleaning and cooking of food and disinfection of food preparation surfaces and related cutlery, serving plates, and utensils. Salmonella food poisoning accounted for over 1 million foodborne illnesses in 2006 and remains an ongoing public health concern for all Americans.

In the case of highly communicable diseases like Covid-19, viral deposition on sink counters, doorknobs, and other commonly touched materials are believed to be a low risk means of exposure. Yet the level of risk has yet to be quantified. Out of an abundance of caution, it is appropriate to wash one's hands whenever coming into contact with commonly touched surfaces. Surfaces exposed to sunlight are far less of a risk than indoor surfaces where sanitation and disinfection controls may either be absent or irregularly performed. The mere contact with SARS-Covid-2 contaminated surface is not a means of exposure if your skin is intact. It is the subsequent hand to mouth transmission caused by sticking fingers in the mouth or nose that creates a potential route of exposure.

In contrast to Covid-19, monkeypox is transmitted through direct contact with fluids or the skin of others infected with the disease. Specifically, monkeypox infects by direct contact with materials that have touched body fluids or sores, such as clothing or linens. It may also be transmitted through respiratory secretions when people have close, face-to-face contact. Washing hands can certainly help reduce exposure but even more critical is avoiding contact with infected individuals or any of their personal clothing or belongings that may contain the monkeypox virus. In this context, handwashing is less important than avoiding exposure to the personal effects of others—whether they are infected with monkeypox or not.

Other diseases that are transmitted through direct contact include chicken pox, hepatitis A and B, herpes simplex, influenza, and measles and pertussis. In many cases, direct contact is not the only mode of transmission but a secondary mode of entry into the body. This is particularly true for the influenza virus that is primarily an airborne pathogen. Exposure to contaminated fomites is also a potential route for influenza exposure—especially for those living in close contact with someone who has already been infected.

Perhaps the most important findings come from a handwashing study conducted to determine the effectiveness of various cleaning agents for hospitals. Handwashing with plain liquid soap for 15 seconds reduced the amount of staphylococcus aureus bacteria on fingertips by 77 percent. Even better cleaning occurred when a 70 percent ethanol solution was used for 15 seconds: resulting in a 99.8 percent reduction in staphylococcus aureus on fingertips. This same study found that even washing one's hands with soap and water for 2 minutes could only achieve an 85 percent removal of staphylococcus aureus on one's fingertips. This underscores the challenges as well as the importance of various handwashing solutions in hospitals as well as in other similar high-risk venues.

The WHO has emphasized the need for improved education of hospital workers, teachers, and students in proper handwashing techniques. A study of twelve- to eighteen-year-old students in India found they were not properly washing hands until shown visual results of what parts of their hands were not being washed. As part of an educational program, the student's hands were air-dried and examined under ultraviolet rays for blue light emission in a dark room. Emission of blue light-highlighted parts of the hands where lotion was still present, and areas not washed properly. Such areas were painted with nontoxic skin-friendly paints. Painted hands were imprinted over graph papers. This visual demonstration resulted in a 73 percent reduction in the amount of unwashed hand area after students were shown where they had failed to wash. The findings of this study underscore the importance of teaching proper handwashing in the public school system. The habits learned while young are carried forward into adulthood. School-going students represent one-third of India's population and therefore their handwashing skills are an important component of any effort to reduce epidemics in India. Similarly, in 2021 American school age children between the ages of five and nineteen represented 19 percent of the nation's population. Their habits will determine the nation's personal hygiene standards in the years to come. These same principles apply in every other nation of the world. Ask yourself, whether you wash your hands for at least 20 seconds as recommended by the CDC? Have you ever been shown the proper technique for fully washing all the exposed skin on your hands? Stopping epidemics caused by food, fomite, and waterborne pathogens starts with handwashing.

## 35.  Can a face covering protect me from epidemic diseases?

Face coverings can protect against airborne transmission of disease, but their effectiveness depends upon several factors. Their value depends on their efficiency rating, fit testing, and the degree of pathogen exposure. Tests conducted on N-95 rated face coverings found most manufacturer's products prevented particles of .1 to .3 microns in size from penetration. The efficiencies of N-95 face coverings increase with larger size viral or bacterial particles with a 99.5 percent protection against penetration for particles of .75 microns or larger.

Mycobacterium tuberculosis can be as small as .65 microns and as large as 7 microns or more. For this reason, an N-95 provides reasonable protection as long as the face covering is properly fit with no gaps. Practicing social distancing improves the value of the face mask. Face coverings even when not meeting the N-95 standard of protection still provide some level of protection particularly for larger droplets coming from a cough or sneeze.

Various levels of more efficient face covering protections are used in hospital settings where communicable disease is routinely a public health concern. However, some of the most relevant data comes from a case study reported by Christoph Josef Hemmer a German physician. According to Hemmer an individual infected with Covid-19 failed to use a face covering on the first part of a bus journey in China and then, prior to climbing aboard a separate bus, donned a face mask. The results follow; as early as March 2020, Chinese scientists described an outbreak of SARS-CoV-2 infections when a passenger infected with SARS-CoV-2, without being aware, failed to don a mask during the first leg of a bus journey. The first leg of the journey took 2 hours and 10 minutes. Of the thirty-nine fellow passengers, five became infected with SARS-CoV-2. During a change of transport, the man obtained a mask. The second leg of the journey, in a minibus, took 50 minutes. During this leg of the journey, none of the fourteen fellow passengers was infected with SARS-CoV-2.

While this case study is anecdotal evidence supporting the value of face coverings, it is important to recognize exposure is based on duration, distance, and dose. It is not possible to tease out the unique benefit of face coverings without considering the following; (1) length of exposure an individual has to an infected person, (2) whether the infected person and the exposed person both wear face coverings, (3) the physical distance separating the infected person from the individual wearing a face covering, and (4) the dose of the pathogen received by the person wearing the face covering. The dose represents the intensity of exposure to droplet as well as aerosol transmission. While all of these variables make it impossible to separate out the unique role played by face coverings, there is strong evidence, when properly worn and fitted they reduce exposure and the likelihood of serious infection. Face coverings do not have to be perfect to reduce droplet and aerosol transmission. This is especially true when other recommended practices are adopted including social distancing and limiting close contact with others to less than 15 minutes. However, if someone should sneeze right in your face and then loudly apologize and continue in that vein for 5 minutes that might be enough to trigger an infection. The key is knowing there are many factors that trigger infection—so reliance on social distancing without a face covering is taking some risk in situation like the one just described.

Bear in mind that it is not necessary to have close contact with other people to catch Covid-19. Covid-19 viruses can remain, both airborne and infectious, in indoor environments for several hours even if the infected person has left the building. In this context, face coverings make sense even if you are the only customer in a restaurant previously filled with infected individuals just before you arrived.

Many Americans found fault with face coverings during the pandemic. At one extreme some believed face coverings were ineffective because the maximum filtration provided might not stop the smallest aerosol particles. At the other extreme some considered face coverings infringements of personal freedom. Concerns with personal freedom were often coupled with the belief Covid-19 was no more serious than seasonal influenza. Both perspectives were reinforced by considerable distrust of government mandates for the use of face coverings. While cloth face coverings provide some benefits the N-95 face mask provides a preferable level of protection for public use—especially when coupled with other personal public protective measures discussed above.

## 36. Which surfaces should be cleaned to minimize the risk of infection, and what sort of cleaning products work best?

The first step in any effort to minimize contact with pathogen contaminated objects is to keep ourselves clean including washing our hands, bathing, and washing the clothes we wear. The world is full of viruses, bacteria, fungus, and other microbial forms of life. Our first line of protection always starts with our own personal hygiene. However, in a highly crowded world in which we share so many common objects with hundreds if not thousands of others, public sanitation and disinfection practices are also essential. Let's review the surfaces that should be cleaned in our home, the public spaces which we normally visit and the efforts to deal with bioterrorism events that raise these concerns to a much higher level of cleaning, disinfection, and sterilization.

Let's start with a review of the objects we might touch if we were visiting New York City for the weekend. Traveling out of our hotel we might touch a doorknob as we exit. Then we push the button to activate the pedestrian walk light. On the other side of the street, we enter a subway where we touch the cashier counter. Then we enter the subway and touch the seat or arm rest. Since the subway is full. Instead of sitting we stand up and grab an overhead strap handle. In a packed subway we might be jostled about and touch someone else's clothing or grab the same strap handle someone else is using and touch their hand. At work we might use a public toilet and then forget to wash our hands. After work we might go to a movie theater, sit down and place our hands on the chair rests. Finally, after the theater we decide to eat at a restaurant serving buffet options. The food is offered on a self-serve basis with common serving utensils. While selecting the buffet option we lean down to get a better look and spontaneously sneeze right on the macaroni and cheese selection. Hoping no one noticed we move to our next selection and use our own fork to grab a potato since the serving spoon offered by the restaurant just didn't work well. If that wasn't enough entertainment for the night, we decide to go to a local fitness center to get a workout. Opening the door to the workout room we find a running treadmill. We put our hands on both hand rests to balance ourselves. As we start walking faster, we exhale at a rapid pace and the speed monitor gets a good blast of our saliva and other particles ejected during our 5-minute run. After our workout we meet a friend and share a cup of coffee at a late-night dinner while sitting at an outdoor table. We share our cell phone with our friend to show a recent newsworthy item. Our friend in turn shows something on his cell phone as well. If you count all the points of contact where we were exposed to potentially contaminated surfaces the results are typical of life in an urban environment. Then count the number of cases where we served as the vehicle for exposing others to our germs.

The purpose of this example is to underscore that many aspects of our daily routines expose us to surfaces and objects that may contain pathogens. Public facilities—whether public or privately owned—have a responsibility to regularly clean objects and surfaces commonly used by the public. The degree to which sanitation and disinfection is practiced is directly related to the health of the public. For example, the standards for sanitation and disinfection must be much greater for hospitals, nursing homes, elderly housing, and for immunocompromised individuals.

Now let's discuss the surfaces and materials within our homes that may cause infection. There are three areas of concern: (1) surfaces and materials that are the reservoirs for pathogens, (2) disseminators of pathogen reservoirs, and (3) food preparation and handling areas. Pathogen reservoirs are associated with toilets, sinks, bathtubs, wash buckets, and drains. All these surfaces are in routine contact with microbial forms of life that can easily release pathogens posing a risk to human health. The second concern is for what are called reservoir disseminators such as wash cloths, sponges, and mops that come into direct contact with pathogen reservoirs within the home. They serve as carriers of disease to other parts of the home.

Finally, the third element of a home disinfection program includes food preparation and handling areas where food contacts cutting boards, kitchen counters, faucets, floors, soiled wash cloths, and various cutlery and serving dishes. If any of these items are not cleaned with soap and water on a regular basis, they can become reservoirs for microbial organisms or serve as pathogen disseminators. For example, mop heads often serve no better purpose than spreading germs evenly around the floor. Similarly, sponges used for cleaning cutlery and dishes shouldn't be used for cleaning bathtubs, bathroom sinks, and toilets. That merely spreads pathogens from one part of the house to another. Using diluted bleach solutions for cleaning floors, sinks and toilet bowls can be useful provided soap and water are used first to remove organic matter. The level of cleaning in the home is normally using soap and water. However, sanitizing products are sometimes used, including diluted solutions of bleach for hard surfaces, such as counters and sinks as recommended by the product manufacturer.

When a home has had a case or cases of a communicable disease, then the standard of care will include the use of approved disinfection products as recommended by the US Environmental Protection Agency. Since there are a wide range of potential pathogens that may pose a health risk, there is no universal disinfection product that works against all microbes. Cleaning surfaces within the home is only one element of a comprehensive approach to avoiding exposure to pathogens. We also must be sure our own body is not a vehicle for disseminating disease bearing organisms. The level of hand cleaning appropriate in the home is normally thorough washing with soap and water for at least 20 seconds. However, if water is not available the CDC recommends an alcohol solution containing at least 60 percent alcohol. For these reasons there is a hierarchy of cleaning strategies reflecting the range of risks and the range of susceptibilities to those exposed. The cleaning methods used must be tailored to the microbial agents that are the cause of concern.

Individuals who work in biosafety laboratories have a much more rigorous procedures for decontamination than those used in the home or hospital. Biosafety labs work with highly lethal pathogens. In these highly secure facilities, lab workers may use self-contained breathing apparatus or similar approaches to decouple their air supply from the zone where the laboratory research is being undertaken. Thorough cleaning is required before disinfection and sterilization. This is because inorganic and organic materials that remain on instruments interferes with subsequent disinfection procedures. Also, if organic materials remain on surgical instruments or other medical equipment and get baked on during the autoclave process, they become even harder to remove later on. Autoclaves use high temperatures and pressure to sterilize equipment. Disposable outerwear is then incinerated to meet sterilization standards.

The CDC has identified several mechanical or automatic cleaners of value in hospital and biosafety labs where the standards of sanitation are extremely high. While you may never have heard of these cleaning systems, they play an important to role when exposure to infinitely small quantities of microbes could be enough to kill you. These cleaners include ultrasonic cleaners, washer-decontaminators, washer-disinfectors, and washer-sterilizers. Ultrasonic cleaning removes soil from cracks, gaps, and cavities of instruments using waves of acoustic energy propagated in aqueous solutions to loosen particulate matter from its bond to surfaces. These innovative cleaning and sterilization procedures are for those working in the highest risk environments on the planet.

In the world of bioterrorism response, the efforts of public health professionals focus on microbial-specific disinfection and sterilization procedures. The most lethal bioterrorism agent in the world is the spore version of Bacillus anthracis, the bacterium that causes anthrax. A review of the disinfection procedures for anthrax provides insights into decontamination methods used for other bio-warfare agents. A variety of approaches are used to decontaminate materials and substances impacted by a bio-terrorist events. The anthrax attacks of 2001 affected buildings, people, clothing, computers, mail, furniture, rugs, and many other non-animate objects. For example, special decontamination procedures were developed for numerous government buildings in Washington, DC, affected by the 2001 anthrax attacks. The US Postal Service, and the US Congress relied on chlorine dioxide gas to fumigate entire buildings contaminated by Bacillus anthrax spores. In instances, where the anthrax spores affected clothing, a 30-minute contact with a 5 percent solution of sodium hypochlorite was used. It was followed by a subsequent cleaning with soap and water. The use of soap and copious amounts of water were critical since the 5 percent solution of sodium hypochlorite (a bleach solution) is quite caustic and would otherwise destroy the clothing. Similarly, other studies have found a solution of sodium hypochlorite as an excellent decontaminant for Bacillus anthracis contaminated drinking water. In some cases, decontamination was needed for crime scene related items such as letters laced with anthrax needed for crime scene evidence. This included decontaminating clothing directly affected by exposure to anthrax spores. In these cases, the CDC recommended a 0.5 percent hypochlorite solution (i.e., one part household bleach to ten parts water). These examples underscore the importance of adopting decontamination procedures uniquely designed for the types of materials, clothing, buildings, food, and water that may become infected.

While household bleach played a prominent role in decontaminating anthrax-infected materials, more recent studies have found a variety of other chemicals that have proven nearly as useful as bleach. These include hydrogen peroxide, ozone, ultraviolet light, ethylene oxide, glutaraldehyde, boiling, and autoclaving. Not all of these chemical and heating solutions are equally effective nor appropriate for all types of materials that might be contaminated. For example, hard surfaces that are heat resistant, such as medical instruments, may be autoclaved at high temperatures to achieve a high degree of sterilization. In contrast, clothing could not be cleaned in that manner. Instead, boiling clothing for at least 30 minutes in a precise solution of bleach at a pH of 7 achieves a high level of decontamination for many types of cloth—but not all clothing. Several decontamination methods may be needed for different materials. Moreover, the effectiveness of any product depends on its concentration, the agent for which it is applied, the duration of the application and other factors including organic matter co-located on the material to be cleaned. The decontamination of materials laced with highly lethal pathogens, including those with bio-warfare applications, is not an activity to be undertaken by anyone other than highly trained professionals. The chemicals used and their application is also regulated by the US Environmental Protection Agency Office of Antimicrobials Division of EPA's Office of Pesticide Programs. For these reasons, decontaminating bio-warfare agents and similar high-risk pathogens should be conducted by individuals trained in chemical, biological, and radiological response.

Decontamination and sterilization procedures are an area of ongoing research that has attracted considerable government investment in the post 9/11 era. The goal of disinfection control programs is to develop the least hazardous and most effective disinfection strategies based on microbial specific efficacy standards. Without such research, public health officials are in a catch-up game; forced to undertake proof of disinfection studies in the midst of a bioterrorism event. Such research is time consuming and requires public investment in a range of disinfection and sterilization procedures. Responding to releases of known bio-warfare agents is not something for amateur pathogen sleuths.

# 37. Does social distancing work to reduce exposure to epidemic diseases?

Yes, social distancing helps to reduce exposure to disease. Social distancing normally refers to physical distancing from other people. However, there are other aspects to social distancing that influence exposure to communicable disease. For example, one's exposure is also affected by use of face masks, face shields, and the angle at which one's face is pointed to others when carrying on a conversation. In addition, social distancing is affected by location, wind direction, confinement in close quarters and by the duration, and dose of the exposure. The ejection of viral or bacterial particles is also influenced by the type of interaction between two individuals. The release of microbial particles varies depending upon whether one is meditating, talking, yelling, singing, sneezing, or coughing. Each of these interactions creates increasingly higher levels of particle ejections. These particles can be released as droplets or aerosols. An extensive number of recent studies have confirmed aerosol exposures created by singers and extremely loud talkers can travel distances far greater than six feet. While normal conversations may not require separation distances of more than six feet, those yelling or singing can eject aerosol particles that can travel as far as twenty-six feet. Small aerodynamically designed viral particles can be carried even longer distances than twenty-six feet under certain conditions. For example, some restaurant ventilation systems may create horizontal air flows. In this scenario, extremely light viral particles less than five microns in size, can stay suspended in air for as long as an hour or more. The lighter the particle the longer it remains airborne.

Regardless of whether the exposure is to a droplet or aerosol pathogen, the duration of exposure plays an important role in determining the infectious dose. The smaller the infectious dose the greater the benefits of social distancing. An infectious dose is that quantity of viral or bacterial particles sufficient to cause infection. An infectious dose is the minimum dose expected to infect 50 percent of the susceptible population exposed. One recent study estimated exposure to 300 to 2,000 virions of Covid-19 would be enough to trigger infection. In another case study, individuals exposed to infected singers for 1 hour received 1,000 virions in an hour. The singing went on for 2.5 hours and many were infected. These infectious dose estimates were developed for exposure to Covid-19 and do not apply to other respiratory based disease. These singers were all closely congregated together and for this reason social distancing was not in play.

In a world where vaccines are not always available or even fully effective, social distancing limits the infectious dose. Most Americans use face masks sparingly unless public health officials declare an outbreak or epidemic. However, for immunocompromised individuals, the elderly and those with co-morbidities—such as obesity, alcoholism, and or diabetes—social distancing measures is a useful routine precaution. Americans have only recently adopted social distancing in public and are still somewhat hesitant to continue doing so. In part this reflects strong peer pressure in a society where exposure risks are not fully understood.

Social distancing reduces the dose and the exposure and for this reason it helps reduce the spread of disease. However, social distancing is only one of several public health strategies needed during a pandemic. A study conducted of state-level social distancing policies found when those policies were relaxed, the decline in Covid-19 cases was reversed. The social distancing measures that were relaxed or eliminated included rules requiring minimum separation of people in public settings, the relaxation of the size of allowable mass gatherings, school and workplace closings, limitations on travel, limitations on service hours and access and use of recreational facilities. Collectively, these public health controls served the broader purpose of social distancing. In this case the pandemic prevention value of social distancing was recognized only after it was eliminated. The number of Covid-19 cases immediately increased after the restrictions were lifted. The findings of this study underscore the value of public health mandates as tools for influencing human behavior—even in a society that is averse to restrictions on mobility.

## 38. Are there dietary and exercise routines that improve immunity?

Nutritional health has clearly played an important role in the long-term decline of communicable disease in the United States. The evidence for the role of nutrition in the decline of communicable disease was well documented over the period 1890 to 1950. Thomas McKeown found improved nutrition was a major factor in improved health which influenced the rapid decline of communicable disease. In the absence of antibiotics and antivirals during the first decades of the twentieth century, the most plausible factor for improved health was access to better nutrition. Millions of impoverished and ill-fed immigrants came to America during the period 1870 to 1920. These individuals had a greater susceptibility to infectious diseases than those in good health and with a better diet.

The diet-immunity connection was not the only factor influencing the decline of communicable disease in this period. Sanitation standards improved and contributed to the decline in infectious diseases. For example, at the turn of the twentieth century state public health departments did an excellent job of raising public awareness of personal hygiene. Washing hands, cleaning floors, and abstaining from spitting in public places were all important public education measures promoted by health departments at the turn of the twentieth century. The state of health of an individual plays an important role in the response to epidemic disease. In the case of measles, the malnourished are more likely to have higher incidences of mortality than social classes with income to afford proper nutrition. The likelihood of death is a serious risk for children with measles living in poverty, with limited access to food, and previous instances of illness and malnutrition. Not every nation has the standard of living found in America.

Nutritional immunology is a developing field of public health and medicine. An individual's nutritional choices influence his or her immunological health. Improved nutrition influences our energy levels that in turn make us more resilient in the face of infection. What we choose to eat can change the gut microbiome and that influences immunity. Nutritional and non-nutritive bioactive compounds—such as pro-biotics—influence the functioning of the gut microbiome as well as both the innate and adaptive components of the human immune system. However, this is not a one-way street. The immune system, in turn, affects nutritional metabolism and needs and can affect the physiological response to food. Diet by itself is only one of many variables that play a role in our immuno-competency.

The linkage between diet and epidemic disease is not well defined. However, there is strong evidence diets can reduce parasitism. In addition, particular diets can affect the gut microbiome and that in turn affects the resistance to parasitic disease. However, these connections are not the same as confirmed causal linkages. How does nutrition improve immunity to disease in general and communicable disease in particular? Changes in gut microbial community composition have been associated with *Clostridium difficile* infection in humans. Similarly, changes in the pH level of the gut influence the viability of some bacteria. The composition and the diversity of the microbiome are influenced by diet and for this reason there is considerable interest in the role it may play in controlling non-communicable and communicable disease.

Lactobacilli bacteria—derived from taking probiotics or eating yoghurt— are thought to play a role in the treatment or prevention of several human infections, including infection of the digestive tract caused by *C. difficile* and human vaginal bacterial infections. While these diseases have not resulted in epidemic scale disease, they are communicable and are a threat to public health. There are strains of drug resistant *C. difficile* that pose a great public health risk in hospital settings. Microbiomes altered by excessive use of antibiotics have selectively promoted the growth of dangerous gut pathogens, like *C. difficile*. When organisms are under stress, it makes it easier for parasites to replicate throughout the body. A microbiome that promotes *C. difficile* results in chronic diarrhea a direct outcome of the long-term use of antibiotics. Antibiotic-induced disturbance of the gut microbiome can be prevented by transplanting microbiome from healthy donors. Despite the apparent link between diet and microbiota composition, a variety of factors such as host genetics, race, ethnicity, antibiotic use, and environmental factors, may also play a role in gut health.

The second concern is whether lack of exercise impacts our susceptibility to disease. It is well recognized lack of regular exercise contributes to obesity especially when coupled with excessive intake of processed foods, sugars, and preservatives. However, the benefit of exercise to counter susceptibility to communicable disease is not clear. Exercise helps to reduce stress and this in turn helps to improve immune response to disease. Moreover, excessive exercise may also have the opposite affect when overexertion stresses the body to a state of exhaustion. Nevertheless exercise, when done in moderation, is an important means of improving health and general vitality.

In contrast to exercise, the practice of the "Relaxation Response" (Herbert Benson, 2000), another modern term for meditation, has also been prescribed as a useful technique to reduce stress. Meditation has been extensively studied during the last fifty years because of its positive effects on stress relief including lower blood pressure and mental calmness. In an age of frenetic mental activity in the workplace and in the world of internet chit-chat, mental relaxation is needed far more than ever. In this context, the relaxation response reduces stress and the inflammatory impacts caused by the fight or flight syndrome. Both the body and mind need rest to compensate for the fast lane activities found in the modern world.

## 39.  When someone in your household gets an epidemic disease, what precautions should be taken?

When a household member is infected with a communicable disease, it is important to identify the disease and its means of transmission. A diagnosis by a physician can provide guidance on the nature of the disease and preventive measures to avoid its spread. At a minimum, some form of isolation will be required depending on whether the disease calls for hospitalization or at home treatment. Under pandemic conditions, hospitals are often overwhelmed, and the only options are either home treatment or the use of emergency isolation quarters such as giant outdoor tents or repurposed indoor sports stadiums sponsored by state public health agencies.

Respiratory illnesses require increased attention to social distancing, the use of N-95 rated face masks for household members and separate sleeping quarters for the infected person. During an in-home treatment regimen, the individuals serving food and cleaning the room in which the infected person resides must provide a high level of cleaning and disinfection in the room used for isolation. For example, soiled clothing and linens must be removed with appropriate disposable gloves and gowns so pathogens are not transferred to the caregivers or disseminated throughout the household. Similarly, the utensils, serving dishes, napkins, and uneaten food must all be treated as if they were pathogen contaminated. Washing and drying of utensils, serving dishes and trays must be cleaned with soap and water to remove organics and then using an approved EPA disinfectant such as bleach for hard surface items. A one-third cup of bleach to a gallon of water can be used to disinfect contaminated surfaces.

During the period of isolation—a period in which an infected individual is considered contagious—there should be no visitors entering the house unless for treatment and medical support by a physician or public health professional. In the nineteenth century, signs were placed on the homes of those with a communicable disease to warn neighbors of the dangers posed by entering the home. While these signs and notices have gone out of favor, the principles behind these warnings remain a concern even today. If someone asks to come into your home when a communicable disease is present, they must be advised of the situation and requested to remain outside. This is more than a simple courtesy; it can make the difference between spreading the disease to others and keeping it confined within one's own household.

Releasing an infected person from isolation should only occur when their symptoms have disappeared, and they have been tested to verify their infection-free condition. Unfortunately, testing procedures may have limited accuracy in determining if the patient is still contagious. For example, PCR tests can identify pathogen material that may no longer be viable, but this does not indicate the material identified is capable of inducing infection. The decision to release someone from isolation must be done in consultation with a physician.

The above discussion of home isolation is an overview of basic public health practices to protect the exposed family members from the infected person. This is an approach that would normally never be encouraged when hospital capacity exists, and medical and nursing staff are available. Moreover, beyond the benefits of professional supervised care, many hospitals offer negative pressure rooms that ensure airborne pathogens are incapable of being transmitted outside of the room where the infected patient resides. The limitations of hospital care were clearly revealed by both the 1917 Spanish flu and the 2020 Covid-19 pandemic. Both pandemics overwhelmed hospital and medical resources and forced public health professionals to adopt the principles of triage. The practice of medical triage is based on the principle of focusing resources on those patients where the greatest benefit can be provided within the limited resources available. Under these conditions home care may be the only viable option when hospitals have insufficient beds, lack staff and limited time to support infectious disease control measures.

The CDC has developed very detailed protocols that apply to the isolation of those with communicable disease in hospitals. CDC has established isolation guidance that covers ten significant managerial responsibilities. For example, administrative responsibilities must address infection control training, hiring infection control personnel, developing infection control procedures and similar responsibilities. Education of hospital personnel is the second critical element to ensure isolation measures are effective. Other elements of the plan include patient surveillance, the use of standard precautions including hand hygiene, personal protective equipment, and cough etiquette. The decision to accept an infected patient into a hospital requires a patient placement procedure. That procedure addresses the use of negative pressure rooms, or in their absence, the use of alternative procedures. Disinfection is also an important element of a robust isolation procedure and must address instrument sterilization protocols, care of the environment through standard cleaning practices for fabrics, linens, and other items that require special washing. In the case of respiratory diseases, hospitals need special procedures to address pathogens transmitted by droplets and aerosols. These are very challenging to control and can be dispersed throughout the hospital if robust precautions are not followed. Finally, hospitals also need to be mindful of procedures to protect immunocompromised patients located near infected patients. This requires the adoption of special infection prevention protocols and patient transport procedures to ensure the hospital can protect its weakest and most vulnerable patients.

In a world in which we are blind to the transmission of viral and bacterial particles that are ten to 100 times smaller than the naked eye can see, the success of any infection control program depends on a coordinated and systematic commitment to patient isolation. Success also depends on a cadre of educated doctors, nurses, laundry workers, food preparation staff, infection control specialists, and even the building maintenance staff managing the temperature, humidity, and air changes within the building.

## 40. What lifestyle choices can improve mental health during an epidemic?

Humans are social creatures and government-imposed restrictions on freedom of movement influence mental health. For example, the widespread use of lockdowns, school closings, quarantines, and restrictions on large social gathering make it difficult to meet for business and pleasure. In addition, during the Covid-19 pandemic many businesses requested employees capable of working from home to do so. The goal was to avoid the spread of Covid-19 during the first two years of the pandemic. Several studies found the consequences of limited social contact resulted in a 90 percent increase in depression compared to the same period prior to the Covid-19 pandemic. There were other adverse consequences as well; an increase in time spent staring at computer or cell phone screens, a reduction of outdoor exercise, and a decline in time socializing (see question 44).

There were many adverse mental health consequences from being pent up indoors. Yet these restrictions were necessary to contain the pandemic. A factor influencing adverse outcomes was not simply pandemic fatigue. It was also a reflection of the pre-existing mental health issues affecting many Americans. A recent study found 36 percent of the depression found during the Covid-19 pandemic was associated with baseline depression that existed prior to the outbreak. In effect, the lifestyle choices made during the pandemic were often influenced by past behavior. This is not to suggest that changes in behavior are unlikely to improve personal mental health. Rather mental health services are needed as a basic component of human health services in America not just during pandemics. The average American is not getting enough exercise, spends too much time in front of a blinking computer or cell phone screen and far less time in productive social conversation with a live human. Sharing love, joy, and enthusiasm with someone else is an antidote to asocial behavior— yet may be hard to overcome for those without the requisite social skills. A Catch-22 if there ever was one. Many Americans have grown isolated with their only friends accessible by the internet or cell phones. When these asocial interactions become the only means of communicating with others, mental health is affected.

The choices available to improve our mental health start with routine exercise of our body, mind and emotions. A 2021 study in the *Proceedings of the National Academy of Sciences* found the risk of depression increased substantially with larger declines in daily active hours of physical activity during the Covid-19 pandemic. Beyond, mere physical exercise, a "whole being" analysis helps address the broader causes of depression. This includes a commitment not just to physical activity, but to mental and emotional well-being as well. Americans spend a great deal of energy developing intellectual knowledge but far less time developing physical and emotional intelligence. Emotional well-being rests on maintaining and improving social relations with family, friends, and co-workers. As social creatures, we thrive and strengthen our vitality by sharing our lives with those we care for. This is not rocket science. Mothers who love their children create the atmosphere for that child's emotional growth. The principles are no different for people of any age; human contact and friendship are fundamental elements of emotional well-being and play an important role during times of stress. Mandatory stay at home orders found during the Covid-19 lockdowns were agonizing experiences for many people.

At the other extreme, humans also need time alone to recharge including getting enough sleep and mental quiet time. It is important to incorporate quiet time into the normal routine of life. Meditation, running, dance, and Tai Chi have each successfully been used to help with depression. Meditation has been used to reduce blood pressure through breathing exercises, and centering procedures for inner peace. In a world of constant stress and never-ending movement, many Americans are living at the limits of their energy levels—and yet may not know how to stop. Today, physicians trained in meditation practice work with a variety of destressing options to address physical, emotional, and mental aspects of depression. Similar improvements in mental health have been achieved through dance and Tai Chi.

Joining a running club, swimming club, or simply finding friends who enjoy walking in nature can do wonders for our sense of well-being. One Japanese study found nature-based therapy involving walks in the forest improved mental health compared to a control group walking in urban areas. The elimination of noises associated with modern technology led to reduced depression for those on nature walks compared to those walking in the city. These self-reported results were most favorable for those with the highest levels of anxiety. Study participants with high anxiety levels had a greater reduction in the feeling of depression after walking through forest than participants with normal and low anxiety levels. Of 586 participants in the study 182 indicated nature walks in the forests reduced their feeling of depression; 347 participants did not feel any change and fifty-six participants indicated increased feeling of depression. These findings underscore the fact that no one strategy for improving mental health is a cure all for all people.

Adopting healthy lifestyle activities improves mental health. Yet that is not enough. Hand in hand with the positive lifestyle choices we must also give up bad habits. For example, stopping the use of alcohol, recreational drugs, or smoking are three choices each of us can make. Breaking habits is not easy, so it is often helpful to make such changes with emotional support from others seeking the same goals; to adopt good habits and drop the bad ones.

## 41. What are trustworthy organizations and sources of information to consult during an epidemic?

There are a wide range of trustworthy organizations responsible for just in time information during an epidemic. For example, those living in an area impacted by an epidemic may need information pertinent to travel, public and personal health, disinfection and sanitation, financial aid, and emergency support among other needs.

The most reliable organization for public and personal health is the Centers for Disease Control and Prevention, known by its acronym CDC. However, the National Institutes of Health also plays an important role since it manages MedlinePlus an important resource center for medical and public health information. During an epidemic access to information on vaccines licensed for use in the United States is available through the Food and Drug Administration.

Your state health department should also be contacted when the CDC or HHS have failed to address emerging diseases in a timely manner. When a novel pathogen strikes any community in America, local, county, and state authorities may often be better prepared to provide immediate evidence-based guidance than public health experts sitting in offices in Washington, DC, or Atlanta Georgia. However, the great virtue of the CDC is that it manages the Epidemic Intelligence Service, a top gun cadre of the world's best scientists and epidemiologists who roam the world to stay on top of emerging diseases. It is hard to find a better team anywhere in the world.

The US Department of Agriculture (USDA) is also a trustworthy organization especially in cases of foodborne and zoonotic diseases. The USDA has programs that address avian flu and bovine tuberculosis. The National Tuberculosis Eradication Program is administered by the USDA Animal and Plant Health Inspection Service (APHIS). In addition, the USDA Food Safety and Inspection Service is responsible for food safety and security and food and waterborne diseases.

During an epidemic many people may wish to travel overseas. International travel restrictions are the domain of the US State Department. It is the most reliable source of travel information, visa requirements, and travel advisories. In addition to the US State Department, the US Department of Homeland Security also plays an important role in regulating border security and immigration issues. The DHS is responsible for inspecting incoming visitors and determining their immigration and public health status. The Customs and Border Protection division of DHS conducts unified inspections of people, plants, goods, and cargo entering the United States. While the health of individuals entering America is the responsibility of the CDC, on a day-to-day basis this work is delegated to the Customs and Border Protection program.

During an epidemic, the Federal Emergency Management Agency (FEMA) provides disaster relief and supports geographic areas where a disaster declaration has been issued. This support includes relief required during epidemics or pandemics. For example, FEMA is responsible for the mobilization of resources to support emergency medical services, mobile hospital units, and related emergency services. Reliable information on emergency resources available during a pandemic starts with contacting FEMA.

The US Environmental Protection Agency's office of Pesticide Programs is responsible for approving the use of microbial disinfectants to reduce or control the risk posed by communicable disease pathogens. This office provides authoritative information on regulated pesticides including antimicrobial pesticides used to decontaminate infected environments.

At an international level, the WHO is an authoritative source for emerging diseases and for the status of epidemics throughout the world. The WHO provides public health recommendations to address epidemic disease. However, it is always best to first check with the CDC for public health guidance applicable to the United States. The CDC is the recognized federal authority concerning public health.

The Association of Public Health Laboratories (APHL) is also an extremely important source of information on laboratory methods, food safety, infectious disease, and public health preparedness and response. The APHL is a trustworthy source of information during an epidemic since they coordinate the state laboratory response network across all fifty states. The APHL also coordinates epidemic response surveillance and tracking. It is the nerve center of the nation's disease tracking system.

Similarly, the American Public Health Association (APHA) is another non-profit organization that has long played a guiding role combating epidemics. Perhaps, one of its most valuable resources is its Control of Communicable Diseases Manual. The manual has been regularly updated over the last 100 years to provide public health and medical practitioners with up-to-date information on the diagnosis, transmission characteristics, and preventive measures for epidemic scale disease. The APHA also publishes, by subscription, the *American Journal of Public Health*.

In addition, there are a wide range of public health, medical, and emergency medicine organizations that provide authoritative guidance on the nature of disease, the modes of transmission and preventive measures appropriate for any given epidemic. These organizations include the National Academy of Sciences, publisher of the *Proceeding of the National Academy of Sciences*; the Infectious Disease Society of America, publisher of the *Journal of Infectious Diseases*; and the American Medical Association, publisher of the *Journal of American Medical Association*. In addition, there are several important subscription-based medical journals that provide leading edge medical research on infectious disease including the *New England Journal of Medicine*, *Lancet*, and *Nature*. These medical and public health publications do not replace the guidance provided by the CDC. However, they are often resources upon which the CDC relies for its own policy decisions.

Several other organizations focus on the occupational and public health needs of specific groups such as epidemiologists. The Council of State and Territorial Epidemiologists organizes conferences and shares information amongst state epidemiologists and therefore is a resource for those seeking to work closely with state-level epidemic response teams. Similarly, the Association of State and Territorial Health Officials (ASTHO) is an important coordinating organization for the fifty states' health officials. ASTHO works closely with the CDC in the development of consistent strategies for public health data collection systems across the United States.

Several government military organizations are important resources for epidemic scale disease—especially those associated with bioterrorism or bio-warfare events. The US Defense Department's Northern Command provides military support to FEMA when medical resources are requested. Similarly, the Defense Threat Reduction Agency is responsible for dealing with CBRNE threats—chemical, biological, radioactive, nuclear—as they impact the United States and its allies. Since epidemics represent a threat to national security the Defense Intelligence Agency also plays an important role in identifying potential biological threats to the United States and the American military. Last but not least, the Defense Risk Reduction Agency is responsible for addressing weapons of mass destruction and this mission includes addressing biological threats. These military organizations focus on emergency response services. Their resources supplement those of the civilian sector and provide information on biological threats to national security. Defense department organizations provide trustworthy sources of information on military capabilities and biological warfare concerns.

# The Impact of Epidemics and Pandemics

## 42. Do epidemics affect certain groups of people more than others?

Epidemics are equal opportunity infectors. However, susceptibility to infection is not equal across all income and ethnic groups. Infectious disease does not discriminate by race, creed, color, religion, income level, or social class. However, these socio-economic factors influence the relative susceptibility, and immunity to disease within the population at large. Poverty plays an outsized role in explaining the greater impacts of epidemics on the poor than the rich. Poverty is highly correlated with overcrowded housing, poor nutrition, lack of access to educational opportunities, and lack of access to public health resources. Overcrowded living conditions facilitate exposure to disease and poor nutrition, alcoholism, and smoking—all of which are influenced by income levels—adversely affect immunity.

The US Census American Community Survey for 2021 found 9.1 percent of all American families had incomes below the poverty level. However, there were marked differences in poverty between white, Black, and Hispanic families. Only 6.3 percent of all white families fell under the poverty level. In contrast 18.1 percent of African American and 15.1 percent of Hispanic families fell below the poverty level. Other factors that influence poverty are household size and the education of the householder. The Census found 23.5 percent of families where the head of household had less than a high school education fell below the poverty level. The most severe poverty was associated with families with five or more children; 35.1 percent of these families were living below the poverty level in 2021. Families with incomes below the poverty level have fewer discretionary funds for education, health care, health insurance, and food.

Efforts to reduce the adverse impacts of epidemic disease must address the root causes of why certain groups are more vulnerable to higher rates of morbidity and mortality. Differential impacts of epidemic-scale disease suggest improved health outcomes during an epidemic require systematic effort to upgrade housing, education, and income levels. Massive disparities exist between the haves and the have-nots. American wealth has never been more inequitably distributed than during the last thirty years. The concentration of wealth in a very limited sector of American society stands in contrast to millions of families barely able to meet basic needs for food, clothing, and shelter. *The New York Times* columnist David Leonhardt declared "the basic problem is that most families used to receive something approaching their fair share of economic growth, and they don't anymore" (NYT August 7, 2017). These economic disparities were amplified during the Covid-19 pandemic. Adults with less education experienced income declines during the Covid-19 pandemic. For example, of those with less than a high school education 23 percent experienced a decline in their income during the pandemic (Federal Reserve, 2021).

Poverty also affects disease exposure. Specifically, those working in the service trades, construction, and similar activities where remote work was not possible had a greater exposure to other people on a routine basis. Increased exposure to others increased the likelihood of contact with infected persons. These are not new issues. Previous epidemics and pandemics that struck American cities during the eighteenth and nineteenth centuries also had severe impacts on the poor. Market people, tradesmen, and laborers could ill afford to flee to the countryside to avoid exposure to epidemic diseases smoldering in urban port cities. These findings were well documented for epidemics in eighteenth-century Boston (Vidich, 2020).

Poverty had a similar effect on Irish immigrants landing in Boston during the period 1846 to 1850. During that period 112,664 passengers entered Boston by sea and 65,556 came from Ireland. As a result of the Irish potato famine those who arrived in Boston were some of the most ill-clad and emaciated souls ever seen by the city's quarantine inspector. Rather than being welcomed with open arms, the city quarantined anyone coming from Ireland in two open-air quarantine facilities located on Deer Island in Boston harbor. One facility was for men and the other was for women and children. The conditions were so appalling that the Irish rebelled at their treatment. Husbands were separated from their wives and children. If that wasn't enough insult, the Irish were forced to strip naked and be deloused using objectionable caustic disinfectants. The food was so deplorable food riots erupted until the quarantine officer realized the city's quarantine strategy lacked basic principles of civility or compassion. Immigrants, by dint of their poverty and ill health, suffered far more than others during the many epidemics of cholera, typhoid, and typhus that plagued nineteenth-century American port cities.

Tuberculosis has had a long history in early America. It was the most lethal disease of the nineteenth century, and its impacts were associated with immigrants living in overcrowded living conditions. Poverty and overcrowded housing in nineteenth-century urban port cities of Boston and New York facilitated an explosion of tuberculosis cases. Tuberculosis is a respiratory pathogen and the slum conditions found in post-Civil War American cities were powder kegs for explosive disease transmission. Fortunately, improved nutrition, better housing, sanitation, and greater access to public education were all factors for its rapid decline in the first half of the twentieth century.

Even today, poverty plays an outsize role in outbreaks of epidemic disease—especially in highly congested nations like India. Tuberculosis continues to affect those in poverty far more than the rich. Studies conducted in India by American epidemiologists found the poor were five times more likely to be infected with tuberculosis than the rich. Factors that adversely impacted India's poor included greater exposure to indoor air pollution and poor health as measured by a low Body Mass Index score. A low BMI is a measure of malnutrition and/or poor diet. It is a consequence of poverty.

In many parts of the world, poverty is also associated with lack of access to clean water and adequate public sanitation. Public water supplies can be contaminated by leaking sewage lines that run in the same underground utility corridors. One would presume, that this would not be possible if water lines were under pressure. However, in many developing nations electricity is not reliable, and loss of water pressure is the adverse outcome. While contaminated water supplies may affect all income groups, the primary groups impacted are the poor. This reflects a bias toward maintaining and improving public investments in sewer, water, and electrical services in those areas where citizens have greater political and financial resources to demand better service. This is called the squeaky wheel approach—those who complain get the better service.

## 43. Can epidemics and pandemics lead to health problems even after they've officially ended?

There can be long-term health consequences caused by infection from a variety of communicable diseases. For example, a study released through the journal *Nature Reviews Microbiology* estimated one in ten people infected with Covid-19 will have a condition called "long Covid." This condition exists when symptoms of the disease last for at least twelve weeks after the initial infection. Symptoms of long Covid include shortness of breath, severe fatigue, brain impairment, or what might be called a brain fog, nausea, and nervous system dysfunction. Those re-infected with Covid-19 are also equally susceptible to experiencing long Covid symptoms. Less immediate consequences of long Covid include an increased risk of cardio vascular disease, stroke, heart failure, and dysrhythmias. Symptoms can last for years. Numerous studies have found multi-organ damage associated with Covid-19. One prospective study of 201 patients found 70 percent of Covid-19 patients had heart, lungs, liver, kidneys, pancreas, and spleen damage to at least one organ and 29 percent had multi-organ damage. Furthermore, there is some evidence socio-economic risk factors such as lower income and insufficient rest in the early weeks after contracting Covid-19 may have a role in increasing susceptibility to long Covid.

Malaria is also a disease that can generate long-term health problems. The parasite *Plasmodium falciparum* can hide in a person's blood stream without activating the immune system and without any symptoms of disease. This results in the recurrence of malaria months after the initial infection. Neurologic defects can occur in cases of cerebral malaria, especially in children. According to the Centers for Disease Control and Prevention (CDC), these defects include trouble with movements, palsies, speech difficulties, deafness, and blindness. Relapses of malaria may also result in severe anemia. This is known to occur in young children in tropical Africa where frequent infections are inadequately treated. These are examples of the long-term consequences of latent malaria within the human body.

Those infected with chickenpox, also known as varicella/herpes zoster, may experience long-term health consequences later in life. The varicella/herpes zoster can reactivate later in life and cause skin rashes, otherwise known as shingles. One of the common complications is chronic severe pain that can last for months. At least 15 percent of the shingles patients have pain that lasts for 90 days after the onset of shingles. Since chickenpox affects nearly 95 percent of all people on the planet, the risks for long-term health impacts are significant. A herpes zoster vaccine has been developed for use in the United States to prevent shingles and is recommended for those sixty years of age or older.

It is also important to recognize that unless the reservoir for a disease is eliminated an epidemic scale disease can go into hiding. In this sense, epidemics and pandemics never die, they merely hibernate. Once the number of susceptible people in any given region reaches a threshold of combustion, an outbreak can occur. However, if enough people are infected or achieve immunity through a vaccine the disease will be unable to spread. In the case of measles, as long as 95 percent or more of the population is immunized human to human transmission is controlled. However, if over time the population of children, immigrants, long-term visa holders, or vaccine hesitant groups fail to get vaccinated herd immunity will decline. The result will be a resurgence of measles.

## 44. In what other ways can an epidemic or pandemic negatively impact physical health?

Epidemics directly affect physical health in several ways above and beyond the illness caused by exposure to a highly communicable epidemic scale disease. For example, during the Covid-19 pandemic many people reduced the amount of exercise and physical activity simply to avoid exposure to other people presumed to be carriers of disease. Going to gymnasiums, swimming pools, or engaging in close contact sports were off limits during lockdown periods. These were not brief lockdowns. Extended periods of isolation negatively affected the physical health of millions of Americans. Indeed, a Harris Poll conducted for the American Psychological Association in August 2022 found 42 percent of Americans eighteen years of age or older skipped exercise or physical activity during the previous month. While all but one state had terminated the emergency conditions by that time, the after-affects of the pandemic were still being felt. Surprisingly, only 13 percent of the 3,192 Harris Poll respondents indicated their health was excellent even though most state lockdown protocols had ended the previous year.

Lack of exercise can aggravate pre-existing conditions for those who have the least robust physical health. For example, the American Psychological Association study found 67 percent of those interviewed had a pre-existing chronic illness including high blood pressure, high cholesterol, depression, arthritis, overweight, diabetes, asthma, heart disease, and obesity. Many of these chronic health conditions are directly related to, or aggravated by, lack of physical activity. Regular exercise can reduce the physical symptoms and consequences of quarantine-driven isolation. Moderate exercise during and after a pandemic enhances the immune system. There is strong evidence that moderate exercise done on a weekly basis improves our ability to avoid the most severe impacts of infection. Exercise is one of the most prescribed therapies whether one is in a state of health or disease.

Lack of access to health care also negatively affects physical health. When hospitals, physicians, and nursing staff are overworked or infected by disease it may be impossible for those with pre-existing physical ailments to obtain treatment. When life-threatening ailments can't be addressed by understaffed and overworked health care facilities, the physical health of thousands of people is affected. It is not merely lethal pathogens that cause loss of life; it is also the breakdown of the public health system during epidemics that affects the physical health of tens of thousands who depend on physicians and hospitals for ongoing care. The indirect causes of ill health attributable to pandemics are not unique to the Covid-19 pandemic. Millions of people died during the period 1917 to 1919 who were never infected by the Spanish flu. Yet the breakdown in the public health system and the lack of medical and nursing staff available due to the Spanish flu were factors in the unprecedented death rates found in that two-year period.

Lack of access to the health care system was not the only factor. A Gallup Poll conducted in December 2021 found the high cost of health care by itself led to an estimated 12.7 million deaths. The survey of 3,905 adults eighteen years old or older was conducted in all fifty states. One in twenty US adults reported knowing a friend or family member who died in the past year after not receiving treatment because they could not afford it. The indirect impacts that epidemics have on the public health infrastructure and the financial well-being of Americans are often as great a cause for the loss of life as the pathogens causing the epidemic.

Similarly, removal of perfectly healthy people to a congregate setting with dozens of other persons suspected of exposure to a communicable disease can often be a formula for spreading disease rather than stopping it. At the other extreme, even if home quarantine is recommended, there is no guarantee the necessary services will be provided by the public health department (see question 39). For the elderly and low-income individuals living alone, quarantine might adversely impact in-house medical, nursing, home care, or meals on wheels services. During a pandemic these services may be functioning at a lower capacity with fewer staff. Indeed, some social service agencies may be unable to provide any services if their staff are sick or told to stay home. These are not hypothetical concerns. Covid-19 demonstrated what can happen to the most vulnerable Americans in the worst pandemic of the last 100 years. Concern for the well-being of these disadvantaged groups is a high priority for public health departments. However, lack of resources, staff and surveillance programs inevitably fall short during epidemics and pandemics leaving disadvantaged groups with limited medical services or access to physical therapy.

Impacts to physical health were not only a concern of the elderly. Children also suffered as well but for entirely different reasons. Extended periods of close confinement amongst couples with dysfunctional relationships were found to cause an increase in intimate partner violence and child abuse during the Covid-19 pandemic. At least one study identified an increase in child abuse cases during the first months of the Covid-19 pandemic compared to the previous year. Lack of access to in person schooling meant fewer means existed to intervene in child abuse cases. Lockdown conditions prevented normal social service and school surveillance systems from functioning properly. Only reports to the police departments served as the only "last ditch" option for parents or friends seeking government intervention in the abusive treatment of children.

The greater separation from close family the greater the physical health impacts including stress, and hypertension—the medical term for high blood pressure. Yet the opposite state, where families were confined together for extended periods of time without reprieve also created the physiology of stress. In this latter case, violence and child abuse were one of the many negative physical health impacts caused by the pandemic. Our physical health is directly connected to our mental health. The inflammatory response associated with the fight or flight syndrome is linked to the epidemic of hypertension in American society prior to the pandemic (Benson, *The Relaxation Response*, 2000). The pandemic lockdown took hypertension to another level.

## 45. How can an epidemic or pandemic affect individuals' mental and social well-being?

Mental and social well-being are affected by isolation. Isolation may take the form of home quarantine for those exposed to a communicable disease or hospital confinement for those infected. Our ability to accept isolation or quarantine depends in part on our perception of the need for this experience. When we experience illness, our willingness to seek help comes naturally. Fighting off a disease for which we have no immunity prompts most people to seek medical help or hospitalization.

In contrast, when we are quarantined simply because someone suspected we were exposed to an epidemic disease, our desire for confinement is far different. Indeed, quarantine, as it is applied in the modern world of public health creates a wide range of emotional adverse reactions. Here are some of the concerns that go through the minds of those held in quarantine. Why am I being confined when I am perfectly fine? Who gives them the authority to hold me for two weeks when I have no symptoms and I can't afford to be out of work? Isn't quarantine nothing more than guilt by association with an infected person?

The person undergoing quarantine will not have the same mental or emotional response to confinement as that same person would have if he or she were infected. In one case, there is no evidence of disease and yet the individual is confined for two weeks—or some other predetermined time. This form of confinement is simply done out of an abundance of caution on the part of the public health department. The health worker seeks to stop the chain of transmission whereas the person quarantined considers it a restraint on personal freedom. The person quarantined may have little interest in the broader public good that may come from his or her confinement. This is especially true when that person is a single mother with a young child to care for. To add insult to injury the mother may depend on her job to make ends meet and a two-week quarantine could be a financial disaster. What if the government is unable to care for her child and pay her bills? These are real issues that rarely get discussed in the media and yet are examples of why quarantine can have serious impacts on the emotional, mental, and financial health of those confined.

Lack of human contact influences our mental and social well-being in several other ways. Humans are by nature social creatures. We flourish with strong social and familial networks. These networks enhance self-confidence, minimize depression, and increase a sense of belonging. Lacking human contact especially that caused by mandatory quarantine orders, creates stress. Our natural fight or flight response when faced with involuntary controls over our movement and freedom triggers an inflammatory response. The result of internalized anger at involuntary quarantine can lead to depression. This in turn can affect immune competency. The longer the confinement and the greater the degree of involuntary control over one's freedom, the more likely mental health will be affected. According to the World Health Organization (WHO) there was a 25 percent increase in the prevalence of anxiety and depression worldwide during the Covid-19 pandemic. A similar survey conducted by the CDC reported 41.5 percent of US adults exhibited symptoms of depression or anxiety in 2021. The adverse physical effects of isolation are not limited to those in pandemics. A landmark study of 7,000 men and women conducted in Alameda County California determined people with limited social contacts were about three times more likely to die during the nine-year study than people with strong social ties.

While lack of social contact can adversely affect social well-being, the impacts are not universal. Similarly, the level of risk any given person will accept is not universal. Some people are better at accepting change and adjusting to new circumstances. An individual's acceptance of risk—in this case the time spent in isolation from one's normal social contacts—influences our ability to deal with long periods of separation. Rather than perceiving lack of human contact as an emotional loss, those with a resilient mental makeup embrace solitude as a reprieve from a life of overstimulation. It is an opportunity to self-introspect and delve into one's own being. Unfortunately, not everyone is prepared to take on such a challenge.

Similarly, there are those who are community oriented that raised their public service to new levels in the face of an epidemic. These are the courageous public health and medical staff who take up the challenge of protecting those in harm's way. These are the special souls that have a sense of empowerment to fight highly communicable disease to save lives. For this group of risk takers and public health leaders their mental well-being draws them toward the good fight. However, even these individuals can burn out if their pace of work exceeds their emotional and physical stamina. The art of pacing one's efforts is a critical ingredient in keeping mentally healthy for those on the front lines of public health. Epidemics also create a common enemy, and this can often lead to dramatic improvements in the sense of community and strengthen commitments to improving the economic and social condition of the most vulnerable segments of the population. In this sense, epidemics represent moments in time that galvanize public support for improvements to the nation's public health system. By finding purpose—whether that be in simply staying alive or fixing our crumbling public health system—our sense of well-being is strengthened. Mental health requires active engagement with the affairs of the world. It is also strengthened when there is a unified community effort to stop the spread of disease and each one of us believes we are all working for a common cause.

The medical research validating the association between immune-competency, isolation and mental health during epidemics and pandemic is relatively limited. However, there is considerable research linking lack of human contact amongst the elderly with declines in mental and physical health and declines in meaningful social networks. Loneliness is more than an absence of social contact. It is also a symptom of internalized stress. A Harvard study that began in 1938, and is still ongoing, evaluated the mental health of 724 students and adults. The researchers followed the mental health of these individuals throughout their lives and found stress and loneliness breakdown mental health. Indeed, the research team concluded loneliness is as dangerous to health as smoking half a pack of cigarettes a day or being obese (Robert Waldinger, The Good Life, and How to Live It, 2023). It is not a coincidence the elderly, including those in nursing homes, were the most adversely affected by isolation and lockdown procedures during Covid-19. The highest case fatality rates during the Covid-19 pandemic were found in nursing homes and amongst the elderly. In America, 27 percent of the elderly are living alone. This condition increases an elderly person's social isolation which contributes to a less robust immuno-competency. The loneliness experienced by survivors of the Covid-19 pandemic affected the vitality of millions of Americans.

Social networks are far more than chances to chat. We gain friendship, love, and support from those who care for us. These emotional links directly bear on our state of mind and our social well-being. Human immunity is not an island limited to the mental health of an individual. Immunity is a shared level of protection especially in those in close familial relationships. Our mental health depends on the health of our relationships and these unquantifiable human connections play a role in how we feel and our sense of vitality. The antidote to pandemic scale isolation is activating and maintaining our familial and social networks through in-person quality time. While direct human contact is critical, in a pandemic that may not be possible when lockdown procedures are in place. Under these constraints, even virtual reality—like zoom meetings and phone calls—are far better than living in solitary confinement. Take a walk, breath fresh air, and appreciate life while we still have it.

## 46. How do pandemics affect the economy, politics, and culture?

Pandemics have had significant impacts on the economies of the world. Public health investments to control pandemic disease outstrip public investments in virtually all other government social services when the grim reaper strikes. For example, more than 100 billion dollars was spent in the first twenty-three years of the twenty-first century to stop the spread of tuberculosis and HIV/AIDS. In 2003, the United States government launched the President's Emergency Plan for AIDS Relief (PEPFAR) in response to the global AIDS crisis. This was the largest public health investment to fight a single disease in world history. This initiative is credited with saving more than 20 million lives, preventing millions of HIV infections, and accelerating progress toward controlling the global epidemic (PEPFAR Report, 2021).

Yet the investments in AIDS research and treatment are close to a rounding error compared to the $5.2 trillion the federal government committed to responding to the public health and economic impacts of Covid-19 in just three years; 2020 to 2022. Within the federal legislative initiatives approved during the Covid-19 pandemic, more than $800 billion was granted to state governments.

At the international level, during the period March 2020 to March 2022, the International Monetary Fund provided over $170 billion in financial assistance to ninety nations dealing with the public health and economic consequences of Covid-19 (International Monetary Fund, 2022). Since March 2022, the International Monetary Fund provided $250 billion on a quarterly basis for ongoing Covid-19 projects to the nations of the world struggling with the consequences of the pandemic. The World Bank also played a critical role in the multi-national Covid-19 response. The World Bank provided an unprecedented $204 billion in financial support to public and private sector clients in the first two calendar years of the crisis. A significant amount of this investment was focused on development and delivery of vaccines throughout the world. Yet these national and international investments are only a fraction of the total economic and public health costs created by the Covid-19 pandemic.

These investments do not account for lost productivity caused by unemployment due to illness from Covid-19 or long Covid. Similarly, government investments do not fully account for layoffs caused by state lockdown orders that shut restaurants, fitness centers, theaters, and convention centers. While funds were made available by the federal government to assist distressed businesses, these funds did not fully capture the lost markets created by businesses shuttered for months on end. Nor do these governmental investments account for non-reimbursable medical costs or increased costs for food and other staples caused by the lack of workers available to perform critical functions in the agricultural, distribution, and processing sectors of the economy.

Past epidemics and pandemics in America have galvanized the political will to strengthen the nation's public health and sanitation programs. For example, the yellow fever epidemics of the 1790s prompted federal legislation creating the predecessor organization to the US Public Health Service. That epidemic also motivated the Fourth Congress of the United States to establish federal authority over quarantine to supplement state-level public health programs. Similarly, the yellow fever epidemics of the 1790s prompted the creation of the first municipal boards of health in America. It was not a coincidence that they were all located in port cities. Yellow fever was an imported disease. This partially explains why the four municipal boards of health were created in Philadelphia (1794), Baltimore (1794), New York City (1797), and Boston

(1799). At the state level the yellow fever epidemics that struck the southern states in the mid-nineteenth century led to the creation of the Louisiana Board of Health in 1855—the first state public health agency in America.

The cholera epidemic of the early 1890s galvanized American support for increased quarantine controls over those entering the United States. In 1893, Congress authorized the president of the United States to halt immigration when there was clear evidence immigrants were bringing cholera into port cities along the eastern seaboard. There was considerable debate about giving the president such power since this was a period when immigration controls were being transferred from the state to the federal government. There were many who opposed the increasing consolidation of public health and immigration controls in the hands of the president, and the US Treasury Department—the agency supervising quarantine matters assigned to the US Marine and Hospital Service. At that time the US Marine and Hospital Service—the predecessor organization to the US Public Health Service—was rapidly consolidating control over the state and municipally managed quarantine stations. The transition from state and local control of immigration and quarantine was hotly debated. Those that recognized the existence of inconsistent quarantine and immigration controls, felt a federal program would be preferable—especially if the federal government picked up the cost of these services. On February 15, 1893, Congress approved the National Quarantine Act. This law authorized the US Marine and Hospital Service to develop a uniform and systematic approach to quarantine working cooperatively with state governments. For the first time in American history the president was authorized to prohibit entry of any person who posed a risk to public health. This law remains the basis for the public health powers vested in the president today. This legislation would not have materialized without the cholera epidemic striking the port cities of Boston, New York, Baltimore, and numerous other port cities. Crisis was a great catalyst for legislative action. It expanded public health powers of the federal government far beyond the limits envisioned by the founding fathers of this nation.

## 47. How do epidemics and pandemics stigmatize certain people?

There are three ways epidemics and pandemics have stigmatized certain people. The first reflects misguided naming conventions for diseases that identify specific people or places on the planet as the cause for disease. For example, Ebola was named after the Ebola River since the first case was discovered near that river in 1976. The Ebola River is in the Democratic Republic of Congo in Africa and therefore continues to have associations with Africa and its people. The Middle East Respiratory Syndrome, also known as MERS, is associated with Middle East nations, especially Saudi Arabia where the disease was discovered in 2012. Similarly, Lassa fever, a hemorrhagic fever named after Lassa, Nigeria ties this disease to over 200 million people living in that nation. The WHO has recognized the danger of stigmatizing people by such names and effective in 2015 it established new naming conventions. The new procedures use names that avoid impacts on tourism, trade, and animal welfare. They are also intended to avoid causing offence to any cultural, social, national, regional, professional, or ethnic groups.

The WHO's naming conventions are a step in the right direction. However, naming conventions have never stopped reporters from tracking down the source of epidemics and pandemics. In doing so, it doesn't take much public imagination to stigmatize certain people as potential carriers of disease simply because they look, act, or are believed be diseased. Based on this simplistic and reductionist logic, these people are not merely avoided but treated as threats to public health. In essence those who look or appear to be from the epicenter of the epidemic are stigmatized. It is crudely nothing more than "guilt by association." Perhaps the best example of the stigmatism that ensues by this simplistic and irrational thinking occurred in California in 1900. The residents of Chinatown in San Francisco were singled out as the carriers of bubonic plague simply because a Chinese ship arrived in San Francisco with cases of plague on board. Based on an overabundance of fear and racial prejudice against Chinese American citizens, the city imposed a quarantine on the entire population in Chinatown. It was one of the most egregious misuses of quarantine powers of any epidemic in American history. Fortunately, in 1900, the US District Court threw out the city's quarantine order as a clear infringement of the rights of the residents of Chinatown. It remains the most famous federal court decision revealing the level of stigma created by irrationally imposed quarantine orders. The case, known as *Jew Ho v. John M. Williamson et al.*, declared the city's mass quarantine order didn't protect Chinese Americans. Rather, the judge found the quarantine increased the risk of spreading the disease by sealing the Chinese Americans inside an infected district.

In contrast to cases where stigma is created simply by public perception someone is a carrier of disease, the third form of stigma is that experienced by those who have become infected. For diseases that leave no outer signs of illness or infection, stigma may be less obvious to the public. However, when rumor mills get going it doesn't take more than a few emails, twitter blasts, or texting messages to cast aspersions on someone who came down with Covid-19, Ebola, or other communicable disease. This may happen even if they have recovered and are no longer communicable. This form of stigma is often hard to identify except if we notice people who used to be cordial and friendly are no longer going out of their way to spend time with us. Even worse are diseases that leave permanent or semi-permanent disfigurement of our face or skin. Smallpox and leprosy are the best examples of the most stigmatizing diseases known since time out of mind. Those infected with smallpox were often covered with pustules over their entire body eventually blistering and leaving the face and skin totally disfigured. The infection sometimes caused blindness. Those who survived the disease spent the rest of their lives in fear of the stigma associated with their appearance. What made this worse for many smallpox infected individuals was the common practice of qualifying the person being discussed not simply by his or her name but with the extra epithet, the one with a "pocks infected face."

Stigma creates division amongst all of us even though we are all equally susceptible to a wide range of communicable disease. Associating places, nations, ethnic groups, or immigrants as the carriers of disease is the functional equivalent of voodoo public health practice. Bacteria and viruses that pose the threat of epidemics are equal opportunity disease communicators. The fact that a disease may be identified as having originated in one location has only one specific public health value; it enables the nations of the world to undertake rapid response countermeasures to stop its spread as close to its epicenter as possible. There is nothing in the DNA of any human that predisposes them, as an ethnic group, religion, nation, or culture more uniquely capable of transmitting disease to any greater degree any other person. We all are capable of communicating diseases transmissible between humans. That is the burden we all carry when we fail to adhere to personal hygiene and the public health measures limiting disease transmission.

# Case Studies

## 1. So Much for the Six Foot Social Distancing Rule: The Tale of a Loudmouth and a Captive Employee

A young man, Theodore White, just got back from a vacation in Turkey and felt somewhat sick upon return to the United States. Despite having a slight fever Theodore decided to go to work thinking his condition was nothing more than jet lag and lack of sleep. Theodore was full of energy and was not accustomed to taking sick days—thinking it was a sign of weakness. Coming into the office he tried to observe a degree of separation from his colleagues. Everyone could tell he was sick, but no one dared to tell him to go home largely because he was the office supervisor. Theodore had a booming voice and even in casual conversation his voice could be heard even by those in cubicles fifty feet away. He spoke to Philip, a recently hired part-time contractor, sitting about twelve feet away. Theodore was enthusiastic about his Turkish travels and told Philip, "I met with many people from China, Japan and Thailand. We spent many hours together talking about international business practices for companies like ours that want to do business in China."

His conversation lasted an hour and because of his loud voice, and phlegm-filled throat his words seemed to carry a spray not only of his good thoughts, but germ-filled coughs. The distance separating Theodore from Philip did not affect Philip's ability to hear the conversation. Theodore's loud voice was not only commanding, but Philip felt intimidated enough not to excuse himself from his supervisor's presence. Listening attentively to Theodore's stories of Turkey, Philip could feel the aerosol discharges on his face even though he was twelve feet away. The office was without fans or ventilation and Philip couldn't tactfully find a way out.

Theodore stayed home for two weeks after his first day back in the office. During the day Theodore only ventured out of his bedroom for the call of nature or to cough up the phlegm that incessantly emerged from his throat every morning. He had a high fever, and his mucus secretions came in different colors—mostly brown, yellow, and green. He recovered after about ten days. Unbeknownst to Theodore, about five days after his conversation with Philip, the part-time contractor got extremely sick and could barely breathe. As a frail sixty-year-old man Philip took extended sick leave. He eventually succumbed to a disease called long Covid and was never able to return to work. Theodore terminated Philip's contract once he could no longer travel to the office.

Upon learning the Governor of his state declared a public health emergency due to the Covid-19 pandemic, Theodore established workplace health policies. He provided reasonable accommodation for two employees with mobility restrictions unable to get to work due to a lack of wheelchair accessible transportation. Both could now work from home. However, the two employees lacked access to internet services in their homes and were given laptop computers so they could continue working remotely. However, Theodore did not pay for the cost of installing an internet router. Two months later, wheelchair accessible transportation was restored but the two employees continued to work from home.

Theodore soon changed the office policies so everyone could work from home. He also declared everyone could come into the office if they weren't sick. His sense of fair play meant the only people who could not come into the office were those known as disease carriers or admitted to that status. How that would be determined was never explained. Theodore modified this highly flexible policy several times including when the governor ordered more restrictive public health policies. Visitors were now excluded from the office and increased social distancing was required both within the workplace and in public portions of the office. The governor left specific workplace protection policies to each organization to determine what worked best. Starting in April 2020 employees could now work from home four out of five days a week. Under the new rules everyone had to wear a face mask in the office and be at least six feet away from anyone else. He also limited the maximum number of employees in the office to four people on any given day. The twenty employees were each given a different day of the week to be in the office.

The rules were again modified when vaccines became available. Rather than require vaccination, Theodore left that decision to each employee. Without knowing who was vaccinated, those in the office on their designated day continued to wear face coverings and observe social distancing protocols. Theodore believed he could not legally determine the vaccine status of his employees. He considered it a privacy matter protected under the Health Insurance Portability and Accountability Act (HIPAA). Caught in this legal quagmire, Theodore let the employees continue working from home four days a week.

Theodore never required employees to stay home when sick. Only when the Governor declared a public health emergency did he issue a health policy and even then, it only addressed Covid-19 and those who might be "carriers." Given the unknown vaccine status of his employees Theodore expanded remote work to five days week. How could this workplace have been more protective of employees?

## Analysis

Being some of the earliest cases of Covid-19, there was no reference point for diagnosing this novel pathogen. One of the two cases could have been prevented if the office had a stay-at-home sick policy. Philip's health was compromised by Theodore's self-centered behavior. Believing staying at home was a sign of weakness, Theodore didn't recognize the life-threatening consequences of his behavior on an immunocompromised older man. Theodore's powerful voice proved the six-foot separation distance, referred to as social distancing did not prevent disease transmission. Simple formulas, like keeping six feet away from others, fail to account for the dose and duration of pathogen exposure. It also fails to consider the distance separating the infected person from others. Combined these three factors created an infectious dose even over a twelve-foot distance. Social distancing—despite its defects—was barely a public health mantra prior to the World Health Organization (WHO) declaring Covid-19 a Public Health Emergency of International Concern. An office "stay at home" policy did not exist nor did one get established during the pandemic. Theodore should have stayed home after his Turkey trip. His behavior affected the health of at least one employee. He also issued health policies that regularly changed making it difficult to stay current with the rules. Ever-changing office policies reflected a failed epidemic response planning process at the state and federal levels. Seat of the pants decision-making ruled.

Lacking consistent health policies meant unvaccinated employees were influencing office policy in the absence of a requirement that employees get vaccinated. It was not possible to come to work without face masks when an unvaccinated employee might be present and be an asymptomatic carrier of Covid-19. Theodore did not understand that HIPAA does not apply to the workplace. It only governs health care facilities. Employers can require employees to disclose their vaccination status as a condition of employment.

Employers can also require proof of vaccination to return to work if applicable religious exemptions and medical conditions are allowed.

Under the Occupational Safety and Health Administration's General Duty clause employers "must furnish to each worker employment and a place of employment which is free of recognized hazards that are causing or likely to cause death or serious physical harm." Theodore's behavior on return from Turkey was not consistent with OSHA's General Duty clause requirements. Theodore also did not keep his part-time contractor after he fell ill with long-Covid. The Americans Disabilities Act (ADA) could have been invoked to allow Philip to work from home under the emergency public health conditions impacting normal workplace employment practices. Similarly, two workers who lacked home internet access could have received reasonable accommodation within the workplace once wheelchair accessible serve was restored. While requiring them to purchase internet access may have been inconsistent with reasonable accommodation standards of ADA, allowing them to work from home was quite appropriate.

Yet Theodore dramatically improved the workplace by creating more flexible work schedules and remote work options than had previously existed. Epidemics tend to change human behavior on a grand scale. Remote work changed from a rare workplace option to an accepted approach for office work across America. Individuals accustomed to hug or shake hands with strangers now either fist bump, or elbow bump to greet another person. While not everyone follows these new rules, they are now considered normal behavior—a major deviation from previously accepted greetings. Similarly, face masks continue to be used even after the pandemic was declared over. This case reveals how personal health is a public good. It also demonstrates how workplace health policies such as stay at home when sick, reasonable accommodation and mandatory vaccine policies can buffer the spread of communicable disease. Without robust workplace safety policies employees can be the conduits for disease and, in some cases, even trigger epidemics.

## 2. Reports of "Mongolian Purple Plague" Spark Riots in the United States

The Centers for Disease Control and Prevention (CDC) issued a proposed rule prohibiting Mongolians and Chinese from entering the United States due to the prevalence of an extremely lethal novel pathogen along their common border.

The pathogen's name had not yet been declared by the WHO, but newspapers called it the Mongolian purple plague due to distended purple buboes observed on those infected. The WHO was not certain what to call the novel pathogen. The first case was found in Zamyn-üüd, Mongolia and reported to the Mongolian Ministry of Health using their Early Warning, Alert and Response (EWAR) system established in 2009 with WHO support. This small town of 11,527 people is on the border with China. It is also 408 miles south of the capital Ulaanbaatar, Mongolia and about the same distance from Beijing, China. The fact that Zamyn-üüd is a border town raised concern among WHO epidemiologists on the pathogen's origin. It may have originated in Inner Mongolia, an adjoining independent state of China. Did the disease originate in Mongolia or had it crossed the border from China? This initial assessment had enormous political consequences for Mongolia and China. The United States was expected to ban travel from one or both nations which could have serious consequences for trade.

The WHO had recently prohibited using names of rivers, towns, or other geographic references in the naming of disease. These new naming rules meant scientists spent considerable time trying to determine if the disease was a viral or bacterial pathogen and what scientific or descriptive name would be most appropriate. DNA sampling had not been available to determine the cause of death, so this delayed the identification of the pathogen.

While these deliberations continued, the American news media learned of the outbreak in Zamyn-üüd. Reporters noted over 90 percent of those infected died in ten days. The symptoms became the lead headline in numerous American papers; "Mongolian purple plague devastating hundreds of Mongolians." Two weeks later the WHO declared the disease to be Yersinia-22. The term Yersinia refers to the disease known as plague and 22 stands for the year it was first discovered. Without fanfare, the WHO posted the scientific name for this epidemic on its internet website. It's efforts to brand the disease using scientific terminology did not garner much media attention. During that two-week period of indecision, the news media, and internet bloggers released photos of Mongolian and Chinese citizens who had contracted the disease. Soon enough a group of Chinese Americans living in New York City were accosted by ruffians pushing and shoving people and yelling "get out of our country." A scuffle ensued between a handful of people. It soon got out of control when dozens of other rioters joined the fray. The police arrived and arrested dozens of individuals—both the ruffians and Chinese Americans who had simply tried to defend themselves from unprovoked attacks.

By coincidence on the day of the riot, the CDC banned travel from Mongolia and China into the United States. The ban took effect three days from the date of their announcement. The final rule was published in the Federal Register, the official publication for legal notices issued by the United States government. Because it is primarily read by government officials, and those doing business with the government, the public was not informed of these travel restrictions. The travel ban allowed Americans of Chinese or Mongolian descent to visit their homeland. However, they would be required to undergo a ten-day quarantine upon their return home. In contrast, anyone from Mongolia or China was prohibited from entering the United States. The ban was in effect for a ninety-day period from the date of the Federal Register notice.

The CDC's travel bans affected the American economy. Thousands of Chinese businesspeople were forbidden from traveling to the United States for this ninety-day period, causing significant disruption to supply chain logistics. The ban also declared goods made in China and Mongolia could not enter the United States without a thorough inspection for rats and rat fleas at American ports of arrival. Inspection protocols called for quarantine of any goods that may contain these disease vectors. The Chinese ambassador in Washington, DC, protested the travel ban and new inspection protocols asserting Yersinia-22 did not originate nor were there any cases identified in China. Out of an abundance of caution, the CDC kept the travel ban and inspection protocols in place for ninety days but did not renew the ban after finding no cases at America's custom stations. What are some of the consequences of the naming conventions used by the news media? Were the travel bans reasonable public health measures?

## Analysis

One of the challenges of living in a world of 24/7 news coverage is the media stays ahead of the deliberative processes of international and national public health organizations. The two-week delay in issuing a scientific name after the discovery of the outbreak meant "Mongolian purple plague" became the media headline that stuck in the public imagination. The WHO disease naming process came too late to change public perceptions. Moreover, even if the WHO could have reacted in a timely fashion with naming Yersinia-22, without laboratory analysis, its scientific name did not alter how some media outlets branded this disease. The first known cases of the disease came from a Mongolian city on the border with China. Both China and Mongolia are known reservoirs for Yersinia pestis. This disease is spread when infected rats or Tarbagan marmots are bitten by rat fleas who in turn bite humans. The high fatality rate suggested this was a pneumonic plague outbreak and therefore was a highly lethal and potentially even a bioterrorism event.

Finding the source of disease means finding patient zero. Yet finding patient zero is often no more than an aspirational goal. It is not uncommon that patient zero is never discovered—leaving epidemiologists to speculate on the origin of a zoonotic disease. As many as 50 percent of communicable disease cases in America are either not reported or misreported. This is one reason it is difficult to identify the reservoir for zoonotic disease outbreaks. This is especially true in nations without a modern disease reporting system.

Epidemic Intelligence Service (EIS) staff at the CDC are trained to quickly track down reported cases—not those that were misreported or weren't reported at all. A cluster of cases exceeding predetermined thresholds signals an outbreak. However, finding cases is not the same as finding the origin of this zoonotic disease.

The CDC's ability to locate the origin of a novel pathogen was unable to keep up with the speed at which the media molded public opinion. Determining the reservoir for a zoonotic disease is a time-consuming affair placing epidemiologists at a disadvantage in a media world that seeks immediate answers to looming epidemics. Another consequence of delay is economic in scope. Americans consume billions of dollars of Chinese merchandise. The travel bans affected thousands of American box stores selling Chinese made goods; this in turn pressured CDC to discontinue the travel ban after no cases were found at American ports of entry. The travel ban was a reasonable use of government authority given the lethality of pneumonic plague and its possible release as a bioterrorism weapon.

Public perceptions of epidemics are also influenced by postings by internet sleuths, many with scientific backgrounds and others without such credentials. These individuals are normally only a few steps behind public health response teams making their own interpretations of epidemics and their origins. Internet era epidemics have created "infodemics." According to the WHO, "An infodemic is too much information including false or misleading information in digital and physical environments during a disease outbreak." In the case of Yersinia-22, media coverage of the outbreak included photos of Mongolians and Chinese with internal hemorrhaging and swollen lymph nodes, known as buboes. This imagery created an atmosphere of fear, and by association, a fear of the people who contracted it. Despite the WHO's declaration that this disease was Yersinia-22, the American public had already fastened upon the phrase "Mongolian purple plague." It was easier to understand, gave a reference to where it occurred, and it rolled off the tongue. Yet this inflammatory news coverage was not only misleading it reinforced the xenophobic views of some Americans. This underscores the challenges of holding the media to their own journalistic ethics. In a fast paced ever evolving 24/7 news cycle where "just in time coverage" often trumps reasoned analysis, "objective reporting" may fall by the wayside. Rather than pandering to baseless innuendoes about the ethnicity of the victims of Yersinia-22 the media needed to be a protector of public health. This meant not publishing news stories that fanned the flames of violence and cultural divisiveness in America. This is a work in progress.

## 3.  A Smallpox Bioterrorism Event Closes New York City and Creates a Public Health Emergency

The state of New York urged everyone in New York City to get vaccinated due to the release of smallpox in an aerosol form in the New York City subway system. This incident soon triggered federal and international involvement. The release of smallpox is considered a Public Health Emergency of International Concern (PHEIC). Officially, vats of smallpox only exist in two of the highest security biosafety laboratories in the world; the CDC in Atlanta and the State Research Center of Virology, located in the city of Koltsovo in Siberia. Because these facilities are considered well protected and smallpox is extremely lethal, its release in the New York City subway system immediately activated the national emergency response plan. It also activated military involvement since smallpox is also a biowarfare agent.

Smallpox was identified by the Department of Homeland Security's (DHS) Bio-Watch program using sophisticated aerosol detection equipment. The Bio-Watch program provides early warning of a bioterrorist attack in more than thirty major metropolitan cities in the United States. The monitoring system detects a wide range of threats using chemical and biological sensor technologies. On a Friday afternoon, April 10, the Bio-Watch sensors identified smallpox. It took about 2 hours to confirm its presence with laboratory polymerase chain reaction (PCR) testing. This immediately set off national and international response measures from the WHO, the US Department of Health and Human Services, the White House, and more than a dozen American military agencies.

The subway station where the sensors identified the pox virus was not immediately disclosed to the public. When the New York Transit Authority announced there had been a release of smallpox somewhere in the subway system it estimated as many as 3 million New Yorkers may have gotten on the subway during the previous 4 to 6 hours. The mayor of New York, in consultation with the Governor of New York, ordered the subway system to be shutdown. The mayor requested anyone who may have passed through the 23rd Street subway station in Manhattan to call an emergency hot line or to visit the New York City Department of Health website. Within 3 hours of the event the city website provided information on decontamination and self-quarantine procedures, and where vaccines would be provided soon. The mayor emphasized "the vaccine protects those exposed to the pox if you receive the shot in the next seven days." The mayor urged everyone to be calm. The mayor also indicated the state department of public health was working with the CDC to obtain sufficient smallpox vaccines from the Strategic National Stockpile for all New Yorkers.

Most people returned to their homes within the city's five boroughs, but an estimated 3 million workers left the city. Their motives were primarily to return to their suburban homes, but many anticipated a citywide lockdown and wished to stay clear of the largest bioterrorism event in the city's history. In this case, flight and not fight was the order of the day. The island of Manhattan is connected to the world through twenty-one bridges and fifteen tunnels. More than 7.6 million subway riders, nearly 1 million train passengers and about 2 million automobiles enter the city daily.

The mayor reminded the public of protective measures to minimize exposure to the pox virus. Yet the city's media failed to mention the dangers of leaving the city without understanding appropriate decontamination measures, self-quarantine procedures and when and where vaccines would be made available. The flight of 3 million people would soon reveal fifty cases of smallpox in the Long Island suburbs and twenty cases in upstate New York villages and towns.

News of this bioterrorism event created an enormous media frenzy focused on the possible perpetrators being Russian and not on the public safety measures that needed to be taken. The mayor's office and the city and state public health departments were besieged with media inquiries. They were also swamped with citizen requests for information and hundreds of inquiries from every conceivable federal agency responsible for bioterrorism response.

The National Strategic Stockpile staff contacted the New York State Department of Health preparedness coordinator to arrange vaccine delivery. In less than three days, late on April 12, New York City received 9 million vaccine doses. Given the enormous challenge of vaccinating anywhere from 2 to

9 million New Yorkers, the mayor of New York City requested the governor to release the New York National Guard's Emergency Medical Technicians (EMTs) to support the vaccination campaign. Unfortunately, that request took several days. The National Guard had already been deployed to Buffalo due to the worst snowstorm in more than fifty years. Five days after the release of smallpox, the National Guard arrived with 2,000 physicians and paramedics. The city had begun vaccinating early on Monday April 13 with only enough staff to handle 50,000 people a day. With 2,000 additional vaccinators suddenly available an additional 200,000 were getting their shots on a daily basis. At that rate, the city calculated it would take 45 days to vaccinate everyone in the city. The New York State Commissioner of Public Health quickly pivoted and urged priority be given to residents who declared they passed through the affected subway station on April 10. This decision was not well received by many New Yorkers who believed they were equally at risk. How could these chaotic events have been prevented?

## Analysis

New York City and the Department of Homeland Security had planned for a possible subway bioterrorism event but did not anticipate the level of confusion or slow pace of activating resources for a city-wide vaccination program. It also failed to anticipate the level of coordination required to work with dozens of local, state, and federal agencies required to complete decontamination of the subway system under a unified incident command system. They had less than seven days to act for the vaccine to significantly lessen the severity of smallpox symptoms in most people. Ideally the vaccine should be taken within three days to prevent or significantly lessen any smallpox symptoms. The second concern was the potential spread of smallpox. The smallpox incubation period can be as long as eighteen days but is typically between seven and fourteen days. Without a real-time vaccination program, infected New Yorkers could begin spreading the disease as soon as seven days after exposure. Time was of the essence.

The city should have mustered vaccinators from Connecticut, New Jersey, and Massachusetts. An all-points bulletin request should also have been made to physicians within 250 miles. Lacking the National Guard for about five days, precious time was lost. Furthermore, vaccine priorities weren't focused on individuals exposed in the subway. The city should also have prioritized vaccine services for the city's most vulnerable including children, the elderly and immuno-compromised individuals. A cordon at all bridges and tunnels leaving the city was never considered. The publicity concerning the release of smallpox triggered a fight or flight reaction amongst city residents. Inspection checkpoints at bridges and tunnels could have stopped outward traffic to ensure those leaving the city understood the risks they may have been exposed to if they had passed through the 23rd Street subway station. While a complete lockdown of New York City was virtually impossible, the outmigration of an estimated 3 million people—many of whom may have been exposed to smallpox—represented a public health disaster that had national and international consequences. Each person leaving the city should have received instructions on decontamination and self-quarantine and procedures for getting vaccinated outside the city.

The media attention given to the bioterrorism event amplified public concern about the dangers of staying in the city. The fact the release occurred on a Friday afternoon when many New Yorkers like to leave the city for the weekend amplified the pathways for smallpox to reach the exurban areas of New York and New Jersey transforming this bioterrorism event from a city crisis to one that affected the entire Northeast corridor of the United States. In the flurry of activity associated with the immediate lockdown of the subway system, the city had not anticipated a smallpox bioterrorism event would ever really happen. It also had not anticipated the mass migration that took place once the public was notified of the smallpox release in the city's subway system. More telling, it had never fully practiced its multi-agency response plans nor anticipated a release inside the New York subway system on a Friday afternoon without the support of the National Guard. It was all too little too late.

## 4. Spreading Monkeypox: The Extreme Burdens of Poverty and Limited Access to Health Care Services

A single woman, named Dorothy Flanders, with a four-year-old child experienced lesions on her stomach. Dorothy had many friends but lived on the margins, relying on housekeeping, part-time writing assignments and occasional waitress work in downtown Boston. Dorothy discovered the lesions one morning and grew concerned if she may have contracted chickenpox or perhaps even Monkeypox, a disease recently renamed Mpox. The news media had discussed a Monkeypox outbreak in New York City and wondered if her close friends from New York may have exposed her during their recent weekend visit to her apartment about seven days ago. Searching for information on her possible infection, Dorothy learned Monkeypox has an incubation period of seven to seventeen days with most experiencing symptoms in about twelve days. Her lymph nodes felt swollen, she had a fever and her stomach rash resembled blisters. It was itchy and she found it hard not to scratch the affected area.

Dorothy did not have health insurance and relied entirely on friends who had internet for her medical guidance. She learned a Monkeypox vaccine was available and could have been used to stop her infection if she had any indication she was exposed. She quickly recognized the absurdity of stopping her Monkeypox exposure with a vaccine. In a perfect world she might have recognized her exposure the previous weekend. Yet her friends made no mention of their infection. Their infection was not obvious when she invited them for a weekend at her apartment. No signs of a rash and no discussion about their health. She was frustrated the Monkeypox vaccine was in short supply even though it was already too late for it to abort her infection. Dorothy's next concern was her young daughter. Reacting to the possibility she might infect her daughter Dorothy consulted with Dr. Alfred Cousy, a general practitioner. Dr. Cousy told her she should check into a Boston Hospital as soon as possible to avoid further spreading the disease. Dr. Cousy was very convincing and gave her a reference to the hospital that evening. After arranging for someone to take care of her apartment she decided she ought to bring her daughter to the hospital since she couldn't afford a babysitter. When she arrived at the hospital, she was immediately taken to an isolation ward. Her daughter was not allowed to stay with her. To make matters worse, the hospital did not provide baby-sitting services for children of hospitalized patients. The hospital said Dorothy could hire an Au Pair or pay for an extended day care facility affiliated with the hospital. Neither option worked since she lived below the poverty level with most of her income dedicated to rent and food. Her friends from New York were not available and for all she knew they may still be infectious. Out of desperation Dorothy found an Au Pair who took her promise of an IOU based on her predicament. Lacking employment with health benefits, this young mother was at wits end in caring for her child.

The hospital staff were sympathetic to her situation, but the hospital's off-site extended day care was for staff—not patients. The two-week isolation period was hospital policy enacted after learning of the spate of cases in New York City. Toward the end of her two-week isolation, she learned the CDC recommended home isolation, an option not mentioned by her physician. If this young lady thought she could self-isolate, she would have done so. The lack of childcare services set her budget back $1,000, roughly the amount she earned every two weeks. Yet Dorothy realized even if she did stay home and self-isolated her financial predicament would be no better. She still needed to keep her daughter isolated from herself while she remained capable of infecting others. Unfortunately, after release from the hospital Dorothy learned her daughter also contracted Monkeypox. Shocked, she pleaded with her physician for advice. This time, he acknowledged the self-isolation option. Despite the onset of symptoms in the young child, Dr. Cousy recommended the smallpox vaccine known as Jynneos, for her daughter since the Food and Drug Administration had approved it for Monkeypox in 2019. He cautioned the vaccine would not stop the infection but perhaps might reduce its symptoms. What should the hospital or the public health department have done to meet her pressing need for family support? How could this crisis have been avoided?

## Analysis

Lacking health insurance this young mother was at the whim of the marketplace. The hospital did not offer extended baby-sitting or day care services and she was not aware of the Child Care and Development Fund (CCDF) that offered childcare support. She also was not aware of the federal and state social safety net services that help mothers with children needing food, housing subsidies, day care services, or income support [i.e., programs such as the Child Care and Development Fund (CCDF), Supplemental Security Income (SSI), Supplemental Nutrition Assistance Program (SNAP) Child Support Enforcement Program (CCDF), or the Rental Assistance Program (RAP)]. Lacking access or knowledge of these programs made Dorothy more vulnerable to Monkeypox. Social safety net programs like SNAP could have helped Dorothy improve her health and that of her child. Poor nutrition adversely affects the immunity of both mother and child. One of the discoveries that explained why epidemics declined in the twentieth century was not because of the development of vaccines—although that was helpful—it was because of dramatic improvements in nutrition and sanitation in America. Being a woman below the poverty level Dorothy's limited access to food and finances brought her close to desperation. Yet her motherly instincts were activated, and she did everything possible to protect her child from Monkeypox. Taking the advice of Dr. Cousy she checked into the hospital only to learn that those without health insurance were not covered for hospital care.

This is a major problem for single mothers without insurance attempting to access the American health care system. In 2021, the US Census found 8.6 percent of all Americans were without health insurance and 11.6 percent were in poverty. However, a staggering 44 percent of single mothers with children under six years of age were in poverty in 2021—revealing the enormous challenges faced by single mothers in America compared to all other poverty-stricken souls who have families to provide financial, housing, and emotional support. Dorothy's predicament is an untold public health crisis that differentially affects the most vulnerable households in America. She was one of 2.2 million single mothers with children under six years of age who were in poverty in 2021. Dorothy's limited financial resources made her far more vulnerable to Monkeypox simply because she was not aware of social safety net programs nor where they could be obtained. Poverty-stricken families and individuals are the most vulnerable segments of our society. They are not well served by the American health care system. Moreover, many of these social safety net programs depend on ongoing federal funding that comes and goes—leaving America's poverty-stricken families to fend for themselves.

What makes this young woman's condition more challenging is that her access to public health information was limited by her high school education and lack of access to digital resources—a common predicament for those who can't afford internet services, cell phones or even cable access to online knowledge. Relying on her physician she took his advice out of an abundance of caution to protect her child. Her child was ultimately infected costing her two weeks of wages and two more weeks of deferred rent payments. Those infected with a communicable disease represent a public health threat to all Americans. Individuals like Dorothy can spread Monkeypox to others if they aren't given the resources to self-quarantine including care for her four-year-old child. America's social safety net needs to be expanded to address this glaring gap in the nation's efforts to control communicable disease. Covid-19 expanded the social safety net during the pandemic. However, many of these programs were cut back—such as the food and nutrition program known as SNAP—after the pandemic was declared over. Yet the need for a public health centric safety net remains as critical for Monkeypox and other epidemics as it was for Covid-19. The health of all people is adversely affected when the most poverty-stricken souls are disproportionately at risk of disease. They are also disproportionately capable of putting others at risk. Fixing the limited public health services available to those in poverty remains a national public health priority.

## 5. Digital Breadcrumbs Expedite Contact Tracing during a Measles Outbreak

Measles cases appeared in a Midwestern town linked to a Columbus Day weekend party. During that weekend dozens of high school and college students arranged for an indoor party in the Buffalo Country Dance Hall located in Deloit, Iowa, a Midwestern college town. Those who attended ranged in age from sixteen to twenty-four. These millennial generation partygoers each had a smartphone with a Global Positioning System (GPS) tracking feature. Wherever these young partygoers went their smartphones knew exactly where they were—a feature that had public health benefits. The GPS applications on their smartphones were accurate within a sixteen-foot level of tolerance. The level of accuracy was also affected by atmospheric conditions and signal blockage issues that often exist in steel or aluminum walled buildings. The partygoers paid little attention to the possible lack of functionality of their smartphone. After all, they were there to enjoy themselves and smartphones were a distraction from seeing old friends who came home from other parts of the United States.

One of the popular individuals who joined the party, Sally Hutchins, had just returned from an overseas assignment to a Middle East refugee camp where she worked for Doctors without Borders. She regaled her friends about the work she did helping refugees who had lost their worldly belongings. These refugees were barely surviving on the rations provided by the United Nations and other relief organizations. She was in high spirits and grateful to be home. Of the forty people at the party, two-thirds came into close contact with her. Sally's charm, outgoing manner, and captivating tales made her the center of attention. The loud band playing in the background nudged her friends closer together to hear what Sally had to say. The party ended at 1 a.m. and Sally went home to her parent's house. The next morning, she had a high fever and noticed small red raised bumps and blemishes on her skin. Not knowing what she had contracted she asked her mother to take her to a doctor—suspecting it may have been related to her work in the Middle East where she had just been eight days ago. The physician told her she likely had measles but out of an abundance of caution based on the rarity of this disease in this Midwestern town, he took a swab sample to confirm the diagnosis using reverse transcription polymerase chain reaction (RT-PCR) test procedures. Within 2 hours Sally learned she had measles. Sally's physician urged her to contact everyone she met since her return from the Middle East. Sally indicated she had exposed her parents and most of the people at the party the previous night. Sally said, "I don't know all the partygoers. I have been overseas for several years and only know about five of the forty people."

Within hours of the test, the state public health department was notified of the measles case by the state public health laboratory. The health department contacted Sally to begin the contact tracing effort but learned Sally could only identify five partygoers. The health department quickly pivoted and requested the United States District Court in Des Moines, Iowa to issue a warrant for the release of GPS data for those who attended the Buffalo Country Dance Venue. The health commissioner declared the warrant consistent with the emergency conditions authorized by the federal Stored Communication Act (SCA), better known as Title II of the Electronic Communication Privacy Act of 1986 (18 U.S.C. §§ 2701 to 2712). Under that law cell phone data must be released "to a governmental entity, if the provider, in good faith, believes that an emergency, involving danger of death or serious physical injury to any person, requires disclosure without delay of communications relating to the emergency." The court approved this novel use of the warrant within 4 hours and the cell phone companies complied with the order the next day. Following the release of the GPS data, the health commissioner's staff identified thirty-six individuals who had attended the party.

Upon being contacted by the health department three individuals were incensed their privacy had been violated. They believed release of their smartphone data meant government officials had access to personal data that could compromise their integrity and privacy. These three individuals contacted their cell phone companies and local government officials, requesting an investigation. They claimed their cell phone data was released even though they never attended the party. They asserted they had attended an adjoining private party that shared a common wall and common air ventilation system with the Columbus Day partygoers. Five partygoers were contacted based on information Sally provided, thirty-three were contacted using their GPS data and phone numbers and two could not be contacted through GPS data. These two individuals were without cell phones at the party but were tracked down through follow-up interviews. What authority do health officials have to access this data? Does this form of contact tracing serve a useful purpose in identifying potential cases of measles?

## Analysis

The health department's emergency use of digital contact tracing relied on the Stored Communications Act provisions authorizing emergency access to private cell phone data when critical for stopping imminent death or physical injury through an outbreak of a highly communicable disease. Even though the GPS data had some limitations on accuracy, it allowed the health commissioner to contact most of the forty partygoers to warn them of their possible exposure to measles. The health commissioner requested each partygoer to contact those people who had been in close contact with them during the previous four days. The public health department had never exercised emergency use provisions of the Stored Communications Act and was apologetic to three individuals who had been inadvertently tracked down.

If this had been done through traditional "boots on the ground" contact tracing the health department would not have reached the partygoers or their contacts within the three-day window where vaccines can prevent illness. The warrant was approved because it did not trigger Fourth Amendment concerns regarding protection from unreasonable search and seizure. This was achieved by limiting the geographic scope of the request for GPS data and phone numbers to those who attended the party and only for a two-week window of time. Despite their outrage at government intrusion into their private affairs, the three individuals in the adjoining party, who shared a common ventilation system with the forty partygoers, were able to receive a measles vaccination three days after the party—sufficient time to prevent infection. However, ten partygoers did not receive the vaccine within the three-day window. They were ordered to undergo self-quarantine for a twenty-one-day period.

In this context, while digital contact tracing expedites the identification of exposed individuals the speed at which post-exposure testing, vaccination, or self-quarantine are implemented represents a continuing logistical challenge for the control of measles outbreaks. Public concerns with data privacy remain significant obstacles to the use of digital contact tracing. Whether digital contact tracing will continue to be used under an emergency public health warrant will depend on public confidence in its value and the degree to which its use is prudently constrained by fixed time and geographic limits on its use.

Fortunately, 300 people who were the secondary contacts of the partygoers got vaccinated within the three-day window from their exposure. In contrast ten of the partygoers were not so lucky. Being beyond the three-day window of exposure where the vaccine prevents illness, the chances for its further spread remained a serious public health threat. Measles can be transmitted four days before the onset of symptoms, so these ten partygoers were potential carriers of disease.

Measles is the most communicable disease on the planet. An infected person can pass the measles virus to as many as eighteen other people who in turn can each infect eighteen more people. Its exponential spread is aided by the release of the virus by asymptomatic carriers. In this context, our normal instinct to take precautions around those who are sick is not activated.

The commissioner emphasized measles is a public health threat in many parts of the country—especially where vaccine skeptics have influenced public perceptions about the benefits of the measles vaccine. He also assured those whose cellphone data had been accessed that the warrant obtained from the federal court for the release of their GPS data—did not include email, text messages, or other communications content contained on their cell phones. The people who were not reached through cell phone data were eventually tracked down using traditional contract tracing procedures—namely through interviews with other party goers familiar with the two individuals that did not have their cell phones turned on during the party.

# Glossary

**Asymptomatic:** An infectious individual exhibiting no symptoms.

**Basic Reproductive Number:** A metric describing the transmissibility of infectious agents. It is influenced by biological, socio-behavioral, and environmental factors affecting pathogen behavior. It is not a measure of disease severity.

**Bioengineered:** Biological techniques to alter or create modified versions of organisms.

**Carrier:** An infected person without symptoms capable of transmitting disease.

**Communicable disease:** A disease transmissible between people or species.

**Contact tracing:** A public health practice to identify and notify those exposed to an infectious disease. Close contacts are notified of potential exposure and of precautions to limit disease transmission.

**Emergency Use Authorization:** An FDA procedure used to expedite treatments during public health emergencies. Unapproved medical products may be used in an emergency to diagnose, treat, or prevent serious or life-threatening diseases when there are no adequate, approved, and available alternatives.

**Fomites:** An inanimate substance such as clothing, furniture, soap, capable of transmitting contagious organisms.

**Immunocompetent:** A person with a normal bodily capacity to produce an immune response after exposure to a pathogen.

**Infective dose:** The quantity of pathogens required to induce illness.

**Isolation:** Confinement of those infected with a communicable disease for a period during which the individual is capable of transmitting disease.

**Microbes:** Microscopic living organisms that are too small to be seen by the naked eye. They live in water, soil, and in the air. The human body is home to millions of these microbes too. They are also called microorganisms.

**Multi-Drug Resistant Organisms:** Bacteria that have become resistant to certain antibiotics making these antibiotics ineffective in controlling or killing the bacteria.

**National Incident Management System:** An organizational structure standardizing procedures to respond to emergencies including epidemics.

**Negative Pressure Patient Care:** Isolation rooms with lower pressure than adjoining rooms that keep patients with infectious illness from transmitting it to others.

**Non-Pharmaceutical Interventions:** Strategies used to reduce transmissible disease including social distancing, face masks, quarantines, school closures, curfews, and similar behavioral measures.

**Pathogen:** An agent that causes disease, particularly viral, bacterial, or fungal.

**Plasmid:** A genetic structure within a cell that replicates independently of chromosomal DNA and is most often found in bacteria.

**Polymerase Chain Reaction:** A quick laboratory testing method used to identify viral or bacterial infections based on small samples of its DNA or RNA genetic characteristics.

**Positive Pressure Patient Care:** An isolation room with higher air pressure than in adjoining areas. Most useful for patients with immuno-compromised conditions.

**Public Health Emergency of International Concern:** An extraordinary public health event posing a risk of international spread of disease. It implies a situation that is: serious, sudden, unusual, or unexpected and requires immediate international action by the World Health Organization.

**Quarantine:** The confinement of individuals exposed to a communicable disease during its incubation period. At its termination an individual will be deemed free of infection or, if not, placed into isolation.

**Select Agents:** A biological agent or toxin which the US government has declared has the potential to pose a severe threat to public health, animal or plant health, or animal or plant products.

**Social Distancing:** Better described as physical distancing, the practice of separating oneself from others (at least six feet). Most useful when practiced in combination with other strategies that reduce disease exposure.

**Strategic National Stockpile:** A national repository of antibiotics, chemical antidotes, antitoxins, vaccines, life-support medications, intravenous administration, airway maintenance supplies, and medical/surgical items that can be requested by state health departments during emergencies.

**Super-Spreader:** An individual who infects a high number of individuals and disproportionately influences the speed or severity of an outbreak.

**Unified Incident Command:** A multi-agency coordination approach, when disparate geographical or functional responsibilities exist, to coordinate incident response with common objectives and strategies.

**Vaccine:** A preparation of a weakened or killed pathogen or component, such as a virus or bacterium, stimulating the immune system through antibody production.

**Vector:** Transmitters of disease-causing organism such as a mosquito or tick.

**Virion:** A complete viral particle consisting of RNA or DNA surrounded by protein shell. It is the infective form of a virus.

**Zoonosis:** A disease of animals or other species that can be transmitted to humans.

# Directory of Resources

## Books

Benson, Herbert. *The Relaxation Response*. New York: HarperCollins Publisher, 2000. A review of the causes of stress and hypertension and behavioral techniques to reduce their impacts.

Block, Seymour S., ed. *Disinfection, Sterilization, and Preservation*. New York: Lippincott Williams & Wilkins, 2001. A reference book of decontamination approaches for bacterial and viral outbreaks.

Cantor, Norman F. *In the Wake of Plague: The Black Death & the World It Made*. New York: Perennial, 2002. The consequence of the plague on the economy and social life of Medieval European Society.

Christakis, Nicholas A. *Apollos' Arrow: The Profound and Enduring Impact of Coronavirus on the Way We Live*. New York: Little Brown Spark, 2021. An analysis of the impacts of the Coronavirus on America and how epidemics impact society.

Covid Crisis Group. *Lessons from the Covid War: An Investigative Report*. New York: Public Affairs, 2023. A summary of the lessons learned from the American government's response to Covid-19.

Gottlieb, Scott. *Uncontrolled Spread: Why Covid-19 Crushed Us and How We Can Defeat the Next Pandemic*. New York: HarperCollins Publisher, 2021. An insider's perspective on the errors made by the American government during the initial response to Covid-19.

Hall, William, et al. *Super-Bugs: An Arms Race against Bacteria*. Cambridge, MA: Harvard University Press, 2018. A review of the increasing threat posed by the spread of multi-drug resistant bacteria throughout the world.

Heyman, David L., ed. *Control of Communicable Diseases*. Washington, DC: American Public Health Association, 2022. The definitive manual on the characteristics and preventive measures for the major communicable diseases that threaten public health.

Hopkins, Donald R. *Princes and Peasants: Smallpox in History*. Chicago: University of Chicago Press, 1983. The classic study of smallpox and its profound impact on civilizations throughout the world.

Horton, Richard. *The Covid-19 Catastrophe: What's Gone Wrong and How to Stop It Happening Again*. Cambridge, England: Polity, 2020. An early critique of Covid-19.

Miller, Joe, et al. *The Vaccine: Inside the Race to Conquer the Covid-19 Pandemic*. New York: St. Martin's Press, 2022. The story of how one Covid-19 vaccine was developed in unprecedented time.

Powell, J.H. *Bring out Your Dead: The Great Plague of Yellow Fever in Philadelphia in 1793*. New York: Time Life Books, 1949. An excellent account of how yellow fever devastated Philadelphia in an age without vaccines.

Quick, Jonathan. *The End of Epidemics: The Looming Threat to Humanity and How to Stop It*. New York: St. Martin's Press, 2018. A review of the causes of epidemics throughout the world and international efforts to control the spread of highly communicable disease.

Rhodes, John. *How to Make a Vaccine: An Essential Guide for Covid-19 & Beyond*. Chicago: University of Chicago Press, 2021. A comprehensive analysis of the wide range of vaccines that exist and how they work and their effectiveness.

Ridley, Matt, and Chan Alina. *Viral: The Search for the Origin of Covid-19*. New York: HarperCollins Publisher, 2021. A review of the controversial theories concerning the origin of Covid-19 and their consequences for stopping future pandemics.

Shah, Sonia. *Pandemic: Tracking Contagions, from Cholera to Ebola and Beyond*. New York: Picador, 2016. An overview of the causes of pandemics including accounts of cholera, Ebola, AIDS, and SARS and how congestion, filth and mobility fuel their spread.

Tierno, Philip M. *The Secret Life of Germs*. New York: Pocket Books, 2001. An excellent account of how germs are spread and the challenges of living in a world filled with microbial pathogens.

Vidich, Charles. *Germs at Bay: Politics, Public Health and American Quarantine*. Santa Barbara, California: Praeger, 2021. A comprehensive analysis of how quarantine and other non-pharmaceutical measures have been used throughout American history including their central role in pandemic response.

Wadman, Meredith. *The Vaccine Race: Science, Politics, and the Human Costs of Defeating Disease*. New York: Viking, 2017. Basic information on the factors that influence the development of vaccines.

Waldinger, Robert, and Marc Schulz. *The Good Life and How to Live It*. London: Penguin Random House, 2023. A unique analysis of how human relationships affect human health and immunity especially during times of stress and depression.

Wolfe, Nathan. *The Viral Storm: The Dawn of a New Pandemic Age*. New York: Times Books, 2011. An account of the search for the reservoirs of emerging pathogens throughout the world as a technique to forecast diseases that have the potential to create pandemics.

# Organizations

### Administration for Strategic Preparedness and Response (ASPR)

https://aspr.hhs.gov/biodefense/Pages/default.aspx

ASPR, an initiative of US Health and Human Services, leads the nation's medical and public health preparedness, response, and recovery from public health emergencies.

**Centers for Disease Control and Prevention (CDC)**
https://www.cdc.gov/about/
CDC is the best source for trustworthy information on communicable disease. It manages the Epidemic Intelligence Service and National Center for Emerging and Zoonotic Infectious Diseases.

**U.S. Environmental Protection Agency's office of Pesticide Programs (EPA)**
https://www.epa.gov/pesticide-registration/antimicrobial-pesticide-registration
Office of Pesticide Programs approves release of antimicrobial pesticides to disinfect or mitigate growth of microbiological organisms.

**U.S. Food and Drug Administration (FDA)**
https://www.fda.gov/vaccines-blood-biologics/vaccines/vaccines-licensed-use-united-states
The FDA is responsible for the review and approval of vaccines, antibiotics, and antivirals released for public use. It ensures vaccines meet safety and efficacy standards.

**World Health Organization (WHO)**
https://www.who.int/emergencies/disease-outbreak-news
WHO is the United Nations agency responsible for coordinating international public health emergencies. It represents the public health interests of 196 member nations.

# Websites

**American Public Health Association**
https://www.apha.org/Publications/Published-Books
An important website to stay informed on public health policy at all levels of government.

**Association of Public Health Laboratories**
https://www.aphl.org/Pages/default.aspx
A valuable resource on the role played by public health laboratories in the control of epidemics.

**Doctors without Borders**
https://www.doctorswithoutborders.org/
An online resource for those interested in the critical role of physicians working on the frontlines of epidemic and pandemic responses.

**Global Polio Eradication Initiative**
https://polioeradication.org/who-we-are/our-mission/
A resource for those concerned about international efforts to eradicate polio from this planet.

**MedlinePlus**
https://medlineplus.gov/
The definitive website to access medical and public health research pertinent to communicable disease.

**U.S. Agency for International Development Global Health Initiative**
https://www.usaid.gov/global-health/health-areas/global-health-security
This website explains the role the United States government plays in controlling epidemic disease throughout the world.

**U.S. Defense Threat Reduction Agency**
https://www.dtra.mil/About/Mission/
Bioterrorism is a national security issue, and this website explains the role DTRA plays in reducing that threat.

**U.S. Department of Agriculture Food Safety and Inspection Service**
https://www.fsis.usda.gov/about-fsis
This website identifies the Food safety and inspection programs of the U.S. Department of Agriculture.

**U.S. Federal Emergency Management Agency**
https://www.fema.gov/fact-sheet/femas-natural-disaster-preparedness-and-response-efforts-during-coronavirus-pandemic
Epidemics and pandemics create a range of public health, housing, nutrition and migration emergencies and this website reviews the role FEMA plays in supporting pandemic countermeasures.

# Index

# About the Author

Charles Vidich, MCP, SM, is an environmental and public health professional with more than forty years of experience in occupational health, bioterrorism response, and sustainable development practices. He served as the incident commander of the Unified Incident Command Center responsible for the federal response to the anthrax crisis in 2001. His extensive experience with large-scale emergency response measures has been chronicled in various books and publications. In 2005, he served on the incident command center team that decontaminated and restored service to thousands of Postal Service facilities struck by hurricanes Katrina, Wilma, and Rita. He is the author numerous books including *Germs at Bay: Politics, Public Health and American Quarantine* as well as numerous publications linking environmental degradation with emerging disease. He holds a United States patent for mercury cleanup protocols. Vidich is a member of the Connecticut Council on Environmental Quality appointed by the speaker of the house. In 2014, the US Environmental Protection Agency awarded him a lifetime achievement award for his work promoting sustainable development.